World Clinics

Pulmonary & Critical Care Medicine

Pneumonia

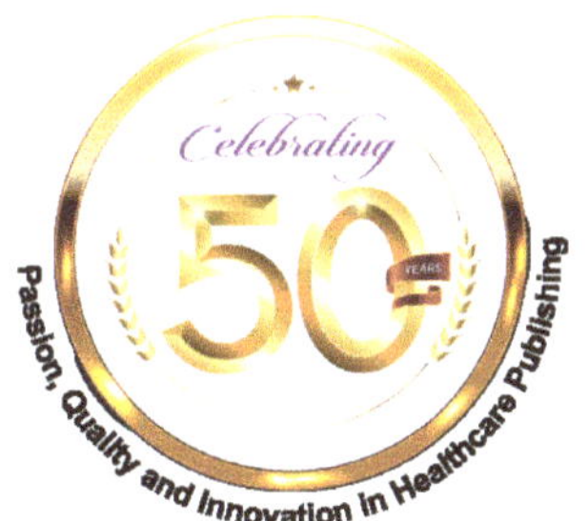

World Clinics

Pulmonary & Critical Care Medicine

Pneumonia

Editor-in-Chief
Surinder K Jindal MD FCCP
FAMS FNCCP

Guest Editor
Ravindran Chetambath MD DTCD
FRCP MBA

2019 Volume 6 Number 1

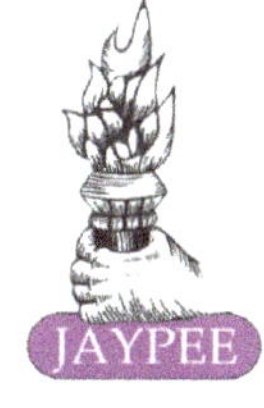

JAYPEE BROTHERS MEDICAL PUBLISHERS
The Health Sciences Publisher
New Delhi | London | Panama

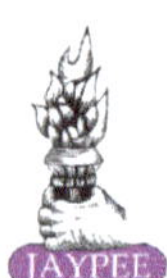

Jaypee Brothers Medical Publishers (P) Ltd

Headquarters

Jaypee Brothers Medical Publishers (P) Ltd
4838/24, Ansari Road, Daryaganj
New Delhi 110 002, India
Phone: +91-11-43574357
Fax: +91-11-43574314
Email: jaypee@jaypeebrothers.com

Overseas Offices

J.P. Medical Ltd
83 Victoria Street, London
SW1H 0HW (UK)
Phone: +44 20 3170 8910
Fax: +44 (0)20 3008 6180
Email: info@jpmedpub.com

Jaypee-Highlights Medical Publishers Inc
City of Knowledge, Bld. 235, 2nd Floor, Clayton
Panama City, Panama
Phone: +1 507-301-0496
Fax: +1 507-301-0499
Email: cservice@jphmedical.com

Jaypee Brothers Medical Publishers (P) Ltd
Bhotahity, Kathmandu, Nepal
Phone: +977-9741283608
Email: kathmandu@jaypeebrothers.com

Website: www.jaypeebrothers.com
Website: www.jaypeedigital.com

Inquiries for bulk sales may be solicited at: jaypee@jaypeebrothers.com

This issue has been published in good faith that the contents provided by contributors contained herein are original, and is intended for educational purposes only. While every effort is made to ensure the accuracy of information, the publisher and the editors specifically disclaim any damage, liability, or loss incurred, directly or indirectly, from the use or application of any of the contents of this work. If not specifically stated, all figures and tables are courtesy of the contributing authors. Where appropriate, the readers should consult with a specialist or contact the manufacturer of the drug or device.

Cover images: (*Left*) The chest X-ray showing opacification of right upper lobe sharply limited by minor fissure due to airspace consolidation with air-bronchogram most likely due to pneumococcal pneumonia. *Courtesy:* Bhavin Dalal, Ishani Dalal, Korembeth P Ravikrishnan. (*Middle*) Coccidioidal spherules in Grocott methenamine-silver stain (magnified view ×400). *Courtesy:* Raseela Karunakaran. (*Right*) mediastinal window of computed tomography showing dense mass like consolidation in UL, additionally LL is also showing consolidation with air-bronchograms (small white arrow). *Courtesy:* Bhavin Dalal, Ishani Dalal, Korembeth P Ravikrishnan.

WORLD CLINICS Pulmonary & Critical Care Medicine: Pneumonia
2019 Volume 6 Number 1
ISSN: 2319-1260
ISBN: 978-93-5270-466-8

Contributors

Editor-in-Chief

Surinder K Jindal MD FCCP FAMS FNCCP
Emeritus Professor
Department of Pulmonary Medicine
Post Graduate Institute of Medical Education and Research
Chandigarh, India

Guest Editor

Ravindran Chetambath MD DTCD FRCP MBA
Professor and Head
Department of Pulmonary Medicine
DM Wayanad Institute of Medical Sciences
Wayanad, Kerala, India

Contributing Authors

Mohan Alladi MD DNB
Professor and Head
Department of General Medicine
Sri Venkateswara Institute of Medical Sciences
Tirupati, Andhra Pradesh, India

Shakti K Bal DNB
Assistant Professor
Department of Pulmonary Medicine
Christian Medical College and Hospital
Vellore, Tamil Nadu, India

Devasahayam J Christopher DNB
Professor and Head
Department of Pulmonary Medicine
Christian Medical College and Hospital
Vellore, Tamil Nadu, India

George D'Souza MD DNB
Dean and Professor
Department of Pulmonary Medicine
St John's Medical College
Bengaluru, Karnataka, India

Bhavin Dalal MD DNB MNAMS FCCP
Assistant Professor
Department of Internal Medicine
Division of Pulmonary and Critical Care, William Beaumont Hospital
Oakland University School of Medicine
Royal Oak, Michigan, USA

Ishani Dalal MD DMRD
Assistant Professor
Department of Radiology and Nuclear Medicine
Henry Ford Health System
Detroit, Michigan, USA

Jyothi Edakalavan MD
Associate Professor
Department of Pulmonary Medicine
Institute of Chest Diseases, Government Medical College
Kozhikode, Kerala, India

J Harikrishna MD
Assistant Professor
Division of Pulmonary Critical Care Medicine
Sri Venkateswara Institute of Medical Sciences
Tirupati, Andhra Pradesh, India

Vivek Jayaschandran MD
Resident
Department of Internal Medicine
Division of Pulmonary and Critical Care, William Beaumont Hospital
Oakland University School of Medicine, Royal Oak, Michigan, USA

Aditya Jindal DNB DM
Consultant Pulmonologist
Jindal Clinics
Chandigarh, India

Raseela Karunakaran DTCD MD
Associate Professor
Department of Pulmonary Medicine
Government TD Medical College
Alappuzha, Kerala, India

M Madhusudhan MD
Assistant Professor
Department of Anesthesiology and Critical Care Medicine
Sri Venkateswara Institute of Medical Sciences
Tirupati, Andhra Pradesh, India

Girish B Nair MD FACP FCCP
Associate Professor
Department of Internal Medicine
Division of Pulmonary and Critical Care, William Beaumont Hospital
Oakland University School of Medicine, Royal Oak, Michigan, USA

Sanjeev Nair MD
Associate Professor
Department of Pulmonary Medicine
Government Medical College
Thiruvananthapuram, Kerala, India

Safreena M Nambipunnilath MD
Assistant Professor
Department of Pulmonary Medicine
Institute of Chest Diseases, Government Medical College
Kozhikode, Kerala, India

Kiran V Narayan MD DM
Associate Professor
Department of Pulmonary Medicine
Government Medical College
Kottayam, Kerala, India

Vijai Kumar Ratnavelu MD DTCD FCCP FAARC FISDA
Professor
Department of Pulmonary Medicine
MediCiti Institute of Medical Sciences
Shamirpet, Hyderabad, Telangana, India

Korembeth P Ravikrishnan FRCP FACP FCCP
Professor Emeritus
Department of Internal Medicine
Division of Pulmonary and Critical Care, William Beaumont Hospital
Oakland University School of Medicine, Royal Oak, Michigan, USA

Rahul K Sharma MD DM
Senior Consultant
Department of Pulmonary, Critical Care and Sleep Medicine
Metro Centre for Respiratory Diseases
Noida, Uttar Pradesh, India

Deepak Talwar DM MD DNB
Director and Chair
Department of Pulmonary, Critical Care and Sleep Medicine
Metro Group of Hospitals
New Delhi, India

Sunny A Thomas MD FAAP
Practicing Pediatrician
Warren Pediatric Associates
Clinical Assistant Professor
Department of Family and Community Medicine
Penn State College of Medicine
Hershey, Pennsylvania, USA

Contents

World Clin Pulm Crit Care Med. 2019;6(1):xi-xii.

Editorial

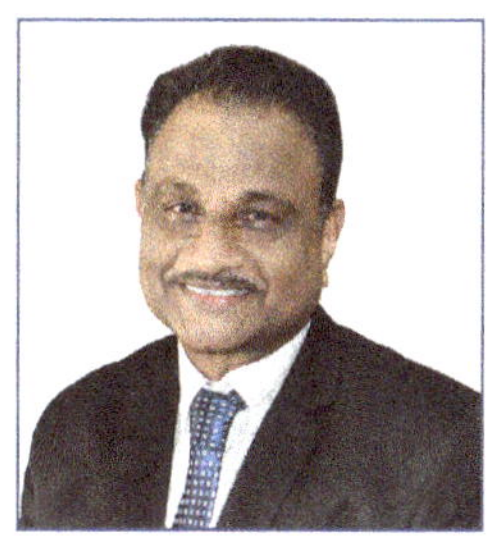

Ravindran Chetambath MD DTCD FRCP MBA
Guest Editor

It is with great excitement and satisfaction that I submit to the readers this issue of *World Clinics in Pulmonary and Critical Care Medicine* dedicated to Pneumonia. This issue highlights the various aspects of pneumonia which will benefit both the students and teachers interested in pulmonary medicine. I have attempted to include all topics related to pneumonia with an international perspective. Both international and national authors have contributed various topics and focus is also given to discuss tropical infections.

Pneumonia has overwhelming importance in clinical medicine and affects all age groups from neonates to the elderly. It leads on to serious consequences such as sepsis, respiratory failure and death. This issue extensively discusses bacterial, fungal, viral, and parasitic pneumonia covering the epidemiology, risk factors, clinical features, and management. Few infections are endemic in certain regions and it is important that this aspect is considered when dealing with pneumonia in those areas. We are also exposed to epidemic or pandemic nature of illnesses such as influenza pneumonia. All these aspects are presented by experts in the concerned fields and I am sure that readers will find it interesting to get updated information on such a common disease. One topic is dedicated to pediatric pneumonia covering its etiology, risk factors, clinical presentation, diagnosis, treatment, and outcome. This is particularly important because pediatric pneumonia differs from adult pneumonia in all these aspects. Newer diagnostic methods including molecular methods are exhaustively discussed and I am sure that readers will find radiology of pneumonia interesting.

My coauthors and I have tried to address some of the aspects of this important disease in a most comprehensive and state-of-the-art manner. I am very thankful to the diverse group of experts who has helped me to prepare this balanced perspective on pneumonia. I sincerely hope readers appreciate and approve our efforts.

Ravindran Chetambath MD DTCD FRCP MBA
Professor and Head
Department of Pulmonary Medicine
DM Wayanad Institute of Medical Sciences
Wayanad, Kerala, India

World Clin Pulm Crit Care Med. 2019;6(1):xiii.

Acknowledgments

I express my sincere gratitude to my Editor-in-Chief Dr Surinder K Jindal who has assigned me the job of Guest Editor of this important issue of *World Clinics in Pulmonary and Critical Care Medicine on Pneumonia*. I am deeply indebted to my coauthors for their patience and sincere efforts to send me the manuscripts in time. I thank all of them for helping me in the editorial work.

I owe much to my wife Reena and my children for their encouragement throughout this work. I am also thankful to my colleagues in the department who has given me free time to complete this project.

I should also thank my publishers Jaypee Brothers Medical Publishers (P) Ltd. and Himani Pandey (Development Editor) for their support and inspiration given to me to complete this issue.

Ravindran Chetambath
Guest Editor

Abbreviations

ACE	Angiotensin-converting enzyme
AIDS	Acquired immunodeficiency syndrome
AP	Aspiration pneumonia
APACHE	Acute Physiology and Chronic Health Evaluation
ARDS	Acute respiratory distress syndrome
ASB	Acid-fast bacilli
ATB	*Aspergillus* tracheobronchitis
ATS	American Thoracic Society
AUC	Area under the curve
BAL	Bronchoalveolar lavage
BTS	British Thoracic Society
BUN	Blood urea nitrogen
CAP	Community-acquired pneumonia
CCPA	Chronic cavitary pulmonary aspergillosis
CDC	Centers for Disease Control and Prevention
CFPA	Chronic fibrosing pulmonary aspergillosis
CFU	Colony-forming unit
CMV	Cytomegalovirus
CNPA	Chronic necrotizing pulmonary aspergillosis
CNS	Central nervous system
COPD	Chronic obstructive pulmonary disease
CPA	Chronic pulmonary aspergillosis
CRP	C-reactive protein
CRT	Chemoradiotherapy
CXR	Chest X-ray
DFA	Direct fluorescent antibody
EBV	Epstein–Barr virus
ELISA	Enzyme-linked immunosorbent assay
EPIC	Etiology of Pneumonia in the Community
FDA	Food and Drug Administration
FNAC	Fine needle aspiration cytology
FOB	Fiberoptic bronchoscopy
GGO	Ground-glass opacity
GM-CSF	Granulocyte-macrophage colony-stimulating factor
HAP	Hospital-acquired pneumonia
HBoV	Human bocavirus
HCAP	Health care-associated pneumonia
HIV	Human immunodeficiency virus
hMPV	Human metapneumovirus
HNC	Head and neck cancer
HSV	Herpes simplex virus
ICH	Immunocompromised host
ICU	Intensive care unit
IDSA	Infectious Diseases Society of America
IFA	Immunofluorescence assay
IPA	Invasive pulmonary aspergillosis
IVAC	Infection-related ventilator-associated complication
MDR	Multidrug-resistant
MERS	Middle East respiratory syndrome
MICU	Medical intensive care unit
MRSA	Methicillin-resistant Staphylococcus aureus
NHSN	National Healthcare Safety Network
NICE	National Institute for Health and Care Excellence
PAIR	Puncture, aspiration, injection and reaspiration
PCR	Polymerase chain reaction
PCT	Procalcitonin
PIV	Parainfluenza virus
PJP	Pneumocystis jirovecii pneumonia
PPE	Parapneumonic effusion
PSB	Protected specimen brushing
PSI	Pneumonia Severity Index
PTC	Protected telescoping catheter

PVL	Panton–Valentine leukocidin
REA-ICU	Risk of Early Admission to the Intensive Care Unit
RSV	Respiratory syncytial virus
RT-PCR	Reverse transcriptase polymerase chain reaction
SAIA	Subacute invasive pulmonary aspergillosis
SARS	Severe acute respiratory syndrome
SAT	Spontaneous awakening trial
SBT	Spontaneous breathing trial
SCAP	Severe community-acquired pneumonia
TBLB	Transbronchial lung biopsy
TLR	Toll-like receptor
TNA	Transthoracic needle aspiration
TNF	Tumor necrosis factor
UAT	Urinary antigen test
VAP	Ventilator-associated pneumonia

World Clin Pulm Crit Care Med. 2019;6(1):1-10.

Epidemiology and Risk Factors of Pneumonia

[1,*]Deepak Talwar DM MD DNB, [2]Rahul K Sharma MD DM

[1]Department of Pulmonary, Critical Care and Sleep Medicine
Metro Group of Hospitals, New Delhi, India
[2]Department of Pulmonary, Critical Care and Sleep Medicine
Metro Centre for Respiratory Diseases, Noida, Uttar Pradesh, India

ABSTRACT

Respiratory tract infections are one of the most frequently reported infections requiring medical attention. Pneumonia is a common and potentially serious condition associated with high morbidity and mortality in all age groups. Pneumonia along with influenza was estimated to be the eighth most common cause of death in the United States and the 7th most common cause of death in Canada. The epidemiology of pneumonia is a dynamic process and has shown various changes in recent years. These changes are due to changes in the population at risk, discovery of new organisms that cause pneumonia, development of antimicrobial resistance, and seasonal variation in the occurrence of pneumonia.

INTRODUCTION

Respiratory tract infections are one of the most frequently reported infections requiring medical attention. Pneumonia is an infection of the pulmonary parenchyma. Community-acquired pneumonia (CAP) is defined as pneumonia not acquired in hospital or a long-term care facility. The CAP is a common and potentially serious condition associated with high morbidity and mortality in all age groups. Impact of CAP is far greater at extremes of age and in high-risk individuals.[1,2] Pneumonia remains the leading infectious cause of death among children under five years of age accounting for 15% of all-cause under 5 mortality in 2015. In a survey by the United Nations Children's Fund, CAP is estimated

*Corresponding author
Email: dtlung@gmail.com

to be responsible for killing 2,500 children per day.[3] In elderly persons also (aged ≥65 years), the incidence of pneumonia is four times greater and associated with more hospitalization and death compared to adult population.[4-6] In this article, the authors review the epidemiology and important risk factors of CAP with emphasis on preventive strategies for the same.

EPIDEMIOLOGY

The overall rate of CAP in adults is approximately 5.16–6.11 cases per 1,000 persons per year; the numbers increase with increasing age.[7] However, the global incidence varies in different studies and different geographical regions based on population and community risk factors. Recent studies have shown that annual incidence of CAP in Europe is between 1.07 and 1.2 per 1,000 person-years and 1.54 and 1.7 per 1,000 people.[8] In United States, CAP occurs in approximately 4 million adults leading to 10 million physician visits, 1.1 million hospitalizations, and 50,000 deaths per year.[9-11] Due to the lack of epidemiological surveys, a clear population-based statistics on the condition is not available from developing countries like India.

The mortality resulting from CAP is high even in developed nations with best of health infrastructure indicating the high lethality of this disease. Pneumonia along with influenza was estimated to be the eighth most common cause of death in the United States and the seventh most common cause of death in Canada.[12,13] Globally, CAP is reported to account for approximately 3.5 million deaths per year and is considered to be highest cause of mortality among infectious diseases.[14] Global Burden of Disease Study in 2010, reported that lower respiratory tract infections, including pneumonia are the fourth most common cause of death globally, after ischemic heart disease, strokes, and chronic obstructive pulmonary disease, and they are the second most frequent reason for years of life lost. Approximately 90% of these deaths are due to pneumonia in people aged more than 65 years.[15] All-cause mortality in patients with CAP is reported as high as 28% within 1 year. As per the World Health Organization, estimated mortality per 100,000 population by pneumonia in India was 89.5 compared to 62 in the United Kingdom and 21.3 in the United States indicating a large mortality burden in lower socioeconomic countries.

The epidemiology of pneumonia is a dynamic process and has shown various changes in recent years. These changes are due to changes in the population at risk, discovery of new organisms that cause pneumonia, development of resistance to old microbial agents, seasonal variation in the occurrence of pneumonia, and increase in the number of immunocompromised patients like organ transplant recipients, number of patients with human immunodeficiency virus infection, patients receiving immunosuppressive drugs for the respiratory and nonrespiratory chronic disease, and association of multiple comorbidities.

RISK FACTORS

Several risk factors for CAP are recognized which affect the disease burden and prognosis. Knowledge about these risk factors is helpful when planning preventive measures to reduce its incidence and impact. Understanding a person with certain characteristics at high-risk of CAP can help to direct that intervention to reduce the risk of infection and impact of disease are targeted appropriately. These risk factors vary depending on the immune status of an individual and include both individual related nonmodifiable factors and lifestyle related modifiable factors along with predisposing host conditions (Table 1).

Age

The most significant and widely reported risk factor for pneumonia is age. With increase in life expectancy, adults aged over 65 years are rapidly expanding cohorts with growth rates almost double that of younger populations. In a report, 20% of the world's population will be more than 65 years of age by 2050. Thus, CAP burden will be even more significant in the coming years.[16] Estimated annual incidence of CAP is 25–44 cases per 1,000 persons in elderly population.[17]

Table 1: Risk Factors for the Development on Community-acquired Pneumonia

Immunocompetent at risk	Immunocompromised at risk

• Age
• Lifestyle
  ◦ Alcoholism
  ◦ Smoking
• Underlying diseases
  ◦ Chronic heart disease
  ◦ Chronic renal disease
  ◦ Chronic liver diseases
  ◦ Chronic respiratory diseases
  ◦ Metabolic disease
  ◦ CNS disease
• Prior invasive pneumococcal disease
• Previous pneumonia
• Other
  ◦ Aspiration
  ◦ Concomitant treatment
	• Immunosuppression
	  ◦ Autoimmune disease receiving steroid/immunosuppressive/biological therapy
	  ◦ Cancer with immunosuppressive therapy
	  ◦ Waiting list for solid organ transplant
	  ◦ Other immunosuppression
	• Immunocompromised
	  ◦ Asplenia/splenic dysfunction
	  ◦ Primary immunodeficiency
	• Human immunodeficiency virus

CNS, central nervous system.

Furthermore, the rates of hospitalization and mortality are also higher in this age group as a result of CAP.[4,18] In an observational cohort study of 623,718 patients aged 65 years or more, it was found that hospitalized rate was 18.3 per 1,000 cases in elderly patients with CAP when compared with four per 1,000 cases in younger populations.[4] The same study showed that hospitalization was even more in adults older than 90 years of age (five times more likely to be hospitalized than those aged 65–69 years). This data suggests that even within the elderly population, those with more advanced age are more susceptible to CAP. This would suggest a possible nonlinear effect, with older age as a risk factor for CAP. Mortality rates in the young patients with CAP are lower than in elderly populations.[17,19] A recent study by Kothe et al., demonstrated that age itself was associated with increased mortality in CAP.[19]

Gender and Race

The results of studies on gender as a risk factor for CAP are inconsistent. Some studies suggest that male gender was a risk factor for development of CAP,[20,21] with CAP incidence and hospitalization rates higher in men when compared to women. In a study done in the United Kingdom, the overall incidence per 1,000 person-years was 1.22 (1.18–1.26) in men and 0.93 (0.89–0.96) in women, whereas men and women aged more than 50 years reported rates of hospitalization for pneumonia per 1,000 person-years of 4.2 in men and 3.4 in women in Denmark.[22] However, these results were nonconsistent in few other studies.[23,24] There is no evidence that ethnicity plays a role as a risk factor for CAP.

Etiological Agent

The potential etiologic agents in CAP include bacteria, fungi, viruses, and protozoa. The true prevalence of the various etiologic agents in CAP is difficult and uncertain identifying etiological agent in clinical practice is difficult. Studies investigating the etiology of CAP by using a variety of microbiological techniques have been performed in different regions and in various patient populations and clinical settings. Most cases of CAP, however, are caused by relatively few pathogens. Pneumococcus has long been considered the major cause of CAP worldwide. More recently, with the introduction of rapid molecular diagnostics, viruses have been implicated to be an important causative agent of CAP along with gram-negative bacteria. Latest and most comprehensive microbiological study of etiologic agents of CAP [Centers for Disease Control and Prevention (CDC) Etiology of Pneumonia in the Community (EPIC) study] done in the United States 2,488 patients demonstrated that the most common etiological cause for CAP is viruses (22%), followed by bacteria (11%), and surprisingly pneumococcal pneumonia was seen in only 5% of the isolates. This changing microbiological pattern could be secondary to development of newer vaccines (e.g., pneumococcal vaccine) and potent antibiotics against bacterial agents, and availability of newer diagnostic tools capable of diagnosing viral pneumonias.[25]

Immunosuppression

An important factor responsible for changing etiology of CAP is the rapidly increasing number of immunocompromised patients including human immunodeficiency virus patients, post-transplant recipients, and patients on steroids and newer immunosuppressive therapy.

This subset of patients has a high risk of developing CAP not only with the conventional pathogens but also with wide spectrum of opportunistic pathogens; furthermore, the presentation may be severe or atypical in this population. List of these newer pathogens is ever expanding but most commonly recognized pathogens causing pneumonia include hantavirus, severe acute respiratory syndrome—coronavirus, human metapneumovirus, *Pneumocystis jirovecii*, *Staphylococcus aureus* isolates carrying the Panton–Valentine leukocidin (PVL) genes, and methicillin-resistant *S. aureus*.[26]

Smoking

Studies suggest that the risk of CAP increases between 50 and 400% in smokers.[27] Multivariate analyzes have shown that smoking has a direct effect on pneumonia onset that is independent of the underlying comorbidities. Quitting smoking is associated with decrease in incidence of CAP by 15–30%. The risk of CAP remains high in ex-smokers in the 2 years after quitting; thereafter, risk tends to fall with years of abstinence.[28,29] The impact of passive smoking is still not clearly understood; although, most studies have observed no significant effect in the overall population.

Alcohol

Other than so many deleterious effects of alcohol, a high level of alcohol consumption is also implicated in increasing chances of developing CAP. A recent study found an increased risk of CAP for men who were heavy drinker (>40 g/day of pure alcohol).[28] Further in the study, a dose response relationship was observed, with no effect observed in moderate drinkers (<40 g/day pure alcohol), even if they are found to consume alcohol daily. In this study, multivariate analysis revealed heavy alcohol consumption as an independent risk factor after eliminating the effects of smoking, chronic bronchitis, heart failure, or chronic liver disease. A similar study in United States cohort also found no association between low or moderate alcohol consumption and CAP.[29]

Environmental Factors

Enough evidence exists on direct effect of environmental and occupational pollution on lung diseases which include bronchitis,[30] bronchiolitis,[31] asthma,[32] chronic obstructive pulmonary disease,[33] and lung cancer.[34] Although all these chronic respiratory diseases in turn increases the risk of CAP, few studies have tried to look at the direct impact of air pollution on CAP. Their results have found soot, crystal silicon, cadmium, and cotton dust itself to be major risk factors for CAP.[33] A case control study concluded that metal fumes, especially iron, reversibly predisposes to CAP.[35] Another study demonstrated that construction and industrial field work (carpentry, painting, etc.) is associated with increased incidence of CAP, as compared to administrative work which was shown to be a protective factor.[36] Despite these few reported case studies, there is no strong literature evidence demonstrating any association between CAP and occupational contact with gases, vapors, gasoline, oil, hydrocarbons, organic, and inorganic fibers or ionizing and nonionizing radiation. An association has been reported between CAP and sudden workplace changes in temperature which was independent of underlying chronic bronchitis and respiratory infection.[34] It is likely that sudden changes in temperature that do not enable gradual adaptation may represent true risk factors for CAP. Further analysis stratified by age showed that people over 65 years of age are more susceptible to this sudden temperature changes.[37]

Sociodemographic

Overcrowding, defined as 10 or more people living in a house, has also been found as a risk factor for CAP. A low education level associated with specific dietary and hygiene habits and conditions that favor the development of CAP has also represented a higher risk for CAP when compared with higher education levels. However, the effect of education is lost once adjustments are made for comorbidity and for occupational status.[37] Married or in a partnership is also found to be a protective factor when compared to single, widowed, or separated. Teenage pregnancy and lack of essential support by health services add to the impact from this risk.

Hand hygiene are long being found as a crucial element in minimizing the spread of most organisms responsible for pneumonia. Simple hand washing with soap and water can reduce the incidence of acute respiratory infections by up to 50%.[23-25]

Childhood Pneumonia

Risk factors for childhood pneumonias are quite varied from those in adults. Apart from the host factors, the incidence is majorly influenced by environmental and family factors. Poverty, poor immunization status, indoor air pollution, overcrowding, and maternal illiteracy appear as the major factors implicated in development of pediatric pneumonia.[38] Malnutrition/poor feeding practices is the single most important factor responsible for significantly increased morbidity and mortality due to pneumonia. More often in these children, manifestations of pneumonia remain occult leading to significantly more lethality.[39,40] Lack of education in parents has also found to be a significant risk factor for both the incidence of childhood pneumonia and as a determinant of the outcome in India.[41,42]

Risk factors pertaining to specific etiologies of CAP may differ from those for pneumonia as a whole and hence, knowledge of risk specific etiology also helps in narrowing down the etiological diagnosis (Table 2). Appropriate antibiotic therapy

Table 2: Risk Factors Pertaining to Specific Etiologies of Community-acquired Pneumonia

Epidemiological risk factors	Associated causative agents
Alcoholism	*Streptococcus pneumoniae*, oral anaerobes, and *Mycobacterium tuberculosis*
Chronic obstructive lung disease	*S. pneumoniae, Haemophilus influenzae, Moraxella catarrhalis, and Legionella* spp.
Exposure to bat a bird droppings, construction sites, caves	*Histoplasma capsulatum*
Exposure to birds	*Chlamydia psittaci*
Exposure to rabbits	*Francisella tularensis*
HIV infection	"Typical" bacterial pathogens, *M. tuberculosis, Pneumocystis jirovecii,* cytomegalovirus, *Cryptococcus* spp., *Histoplasma* spp., *Coccidioides* spp.
Travel to desert, Southwest United States	*Coccidioides* spp., hantavirus (Sin Nombre virus)
Farm exposure	*Coxiella burnetii* (animals), *Aspergillus* spp. (barns, hay)
Postinfluenza	*S. pneumoniae, S. aureus, Streptococcus pyogenes,* and *H. influenzae*

Continued

Continued

Table 2: Risk Factors Pertaining to Specific Etiologies of Community-acquired Pneumonia

Epidemiological risk factors	Associated causative agents
Aspiration	Mixed aerobic, anaerobic
Marijuana smoking	*Aspergillus* spp.
Anatomic abnormality of lung parenchyma, e.g., bronchiectasis, cystic fibrosis	*Pseudomonas aeruginosa, Burkholderia cepacia,* and *S. aureus*
Injection drug use	*S. aureus,* anaerobes, *M. tuberculosis*, and *S. pneumoniae*
Obstruction of large airway	Anaerobes, *S. pneumoniae, H. influenzae,* and *S. aureus*
Incarceration	*M. tuberculosis*
Neutropenia	*Aspergillus* spp., zygomycetes
Asplenia	*S. pneumoniae, H. influenzae*

can be instituted if the exposure and possible clue to causative microorganisms is identified in the history. A possible correlation between various epidemiologic factors and bacteriological cause of CAP shown in table 2.[43] Patient at risk of aspiration like patients of gingivitis and an unprotected airway commonly seen in patients with alcohol or drug overdose or a seizure disorder, anaerobes play a significant role. Anaerobic pneumonias are often complicated by abscess formation and significant empyema or parapneumonic effusions. In hospitalized patient with CAP, atypical bacteria like *M. pneumonia* and *Legionella* spp. have also been detected in approximately 3–15% using nonserological techniques. *Staphylococcus aureus* and *Pseudomonas aeruginosa* are important etiological agents in patients with structural lung disease.[26]

CONCLUSION

Changes in the epidemiology of pathogens due to emergence of new pathogens and changing antimicrobial susceptibility of old ones, difficulty in making an etiologic diagnosis due to limited laboratory methods with low diagnostic yield, and complex pneumonia management guidelines make CAP a unique challenge for the physicians. The thorough knowledge of changing local and worldwide epidemiology, and risk factors, therefore, have implications on planning, further management strategies, and guideline protocols for CAP.

Editor's Comment

Pneumonia is a common and potentially serious illness. It is associated with considerable morbidity and mortality, particularly in extremes of ages and those with significant comorbidities. An important reason for the increased mortality is the influence of pneumonia on chronic diseases, along with the increasing age of the population as well as virulence factors of the causative microorganisms. Respiratory viruses are considered the etiological agent in almost one-third of cases of community-acquired pneumonia. Influenza virus is usually self-limiting but severe complications can occur, particularly in high-risk individuals such as elderly patients with comorbidities or immunosuppressed patients. The choice of treatment is dependent on many factors. These include the setting in which pneumonia developed comorbid illnesses, severity of pneumonia, likely pathogen and likely sensitivity pattern of organisms. It is therefore important to have epidemiological data to guide us as to the likely pathogen that commonly cause pneumonia in our community or hospital setting. Epidemiological surveillance is all the more important to know the new and emerging pathogens causing pneumonia. Authors in this article clearly described the various epidemiological and risk factors in the causation of pneumonia.

Ravindran Chetambath

REFERENCES

1. Welte T, Torres A, Nathwani D. Clinical and economic burden of community-acquired pneumonia among adults in Europe. *Thorax.* 2012;67:71-9.
2. Blasi F, Mantero M, Santus P, et al. Understanding the burden of pneumococcal disease in adults. *Clin Microbiol Infect.* 2012;18:1-8.
3. UNICEF, one is too many: Ending child deaths from pneumonia and diarrhoea. New York; UNICEF, 2016.
4. Kaplan V, Angus DC, Griffin MF, et al. Hospitalized community-acquired pneumonia in the elderly: Age- and sex-related patterns of care and outcome in the United States. *Am J Respir Crit Care Med.* 2002;165(6): 766-72.
5. Fine MJ, Smith MA, Carson CA, et al. Prognosis and outcomes of patients with community acquire pneumonia. A meta-analysis. *JAMA.* 1996;275(2):134-41.
6. Chong CP, Street PR. Pneumonia in the elderly: A review of the epidemiology, pathogenesis microbiology, and clinical features. *South Med J.* 2008;101(11):1141-45.
7. Marrie TJ, Huang JQ. Epidemiology of community-acquired pneumonia in Edmonton, Alberta: An emergency department-based study. *Can Respir J.* 2005;12(3):139-42.
8. Torres A, Peetermans WE, Viegi G, et al. Risk factors for community-acquired pneumonia in adults in Europe: A literature review. *Thorax.* 2013;68:1057-65.
9. Minino AM, Murphy SL, Xu J, et al. Deaths: final data for 2008. *Natl Vital Stat Rep.* 2011;59:1-126.
10. Hall MJ, DeFrances CJ, Williams SN, et al. National Hospital Discharge Survey: 2007 summary. *Natl Health Stat Report.* 2010;(29):1-20, 24.
11. Grossman RF, Rotschafer JC, Tan JS. Antimicrobial treatment of lower respiratory tract infections in the hospital setting. *Am J Med.* 2005;118(7A):29S-38s.

12. File TM Jr, Marrie TJ. Burden of community-acquired pneumonia in North American adults. *Postgrad Med.* 2010;122:130-41.
13. Kung HC, Hoyert DL, Xu J, et al. Deaths: Final data for 2005. *Natl Vital Stat Rep.* 2008;56:1-20.
14. Marrie TJ. Acute bronchitis and community acquired pneumonia. Fishman's Pulmonary diseases and disorders, 5th edition, 2015.
15. European commission. Health Statistics. Atlas on mortality in European Union. Luxembourg: Office for Official publications of the European Communities, 2008.
16. Donowitz GR, Cox HL. Bacterial community-acquired pneumonia in older patients. *Clin Geriatr Med.* 2007;23(3):515-34.
17. Janssens JP, Krause KH. Pneumonia in the very old. *Lancet Infect Dis.* 2004;4(2):112-24.
18. Fine MJ, Smith MA, Carson CA, et al. Prognosis and outcomes of patients with community acquired pneumonia: A meta-analysis. *JAMA.* 1996;275(2):134-41.
19. Kothe H, Bauer T, Marre R, et al. Outcome of community-acquired pneumonia: Influence of age, residence status and antimicrobial treatment. *Eur Respir J.* 2008;32(1):139-46.
20. Jackson ML, Neuzil KM, Thompson WW, et al. The burden of community-acquired pneumonia in seniors: Results of a population-based study. *Clin Infect Dis.* 2004;39:1642-50.
21. Vila-Corcoles A, Ochoa-Gondar O, Rodriguez-Blanco T, et al. Epidemiology of community-acquired pneumonia in older adults: A population-based study. *Respir Med.* 2009;103:309-16.
22. Rodriguez LA, Ruigomez A, Wallander MA, et al. Acid-suppressive drugs and community-acquired pneumonia. *Epidemiology.* 2009;20:800-6.
23. Koivula I, Sten M, Mäkelä PH. Risk factors for pneumonia in the elderly. Am J Med. 1994;96:313-20.
24. Gau JT, Acharya U, Khan S, et al. Pharmacotherapy and the risk for community-acquired pneumonia. *BMC Geriatr.* 2010;10:45.
25. Jain S, Self WH, Wunderink RG, et al. Community-acquired pneumonia requiring hospitalization among U.S. adults. *N Engl J Med.* 2015;373:415-27.
26. Mandell LA, Wunderink R. Pneumonia. Harrison's principles of internal medicine, 17th edition, 2008.
27. Almirall J, González CA, Balanzó X, et al. Proportion of community-acquired pneumonia cases attributable to tobacco smoking. *Chest.* 1999;116:375-79.
28. Almirall J, Bolíbar I, Balanzó X, et al. Risk factors for community-acquired pneumonia in adults: A population-based case-control study. *Eur Respir J.* 1999;13:349-55.
29. Baik I, Curhan GC, Rimm EB, et al. A prospective study of age and lifestyle factors in relation to community-acquired pneumonia in US men and women. *Arch Intern Med.* 2000;160:3082-88.
30. Fishwick D, Bradshaw LM, D'Souza W, et al. Chronic bronchitis, shortness of breath, and airway obstruction by occupation in New Zealand. *Am J Respir Crit Care Med.* 1997;156:1440-46.
31. Wright JL. Inhalational lung injury causing bronchiolitis. *Clin Chest Med.* 1993;14:635-44.
32. Chan-Yeung M, Malo JL. Aetiological agents in occupational asthma. *Eur Respir J.* 1994;7:346-71.
33. Hendrick DJ. Occupational and chronic obstructive pulmonary disease (COPD). *Thorax.* 1996;51:947-55.
34. Steenland K, Loomis D, Shy C, et al. Review of occupational lung carcinogens. *Am J Ind Med.* 1996;29:474-90.
35. Palmer KT, Poole J, Ayres JG, et al. Exposure to metal fume and infectious pneumonia. *Am J Epidemiol.* 2003;157:227-33.
36. Almirall J, Serra-Prat M, Bolíbar I, et al. Relación de las profesiones y las condiciones laborales con la neumonía adquirida en la comunidad. *Arch Bronconeumol.* 2015;51:627-31.
37. Almirall J, Bolíbar I, Serra-Prat M, et al. New evidence of risk factors for community-acquired pneumonia: A population-based study. *Eur Respir J.* 2008;31:1274-84.
38. Ebbert JO, Croghan IT, Schroeder DR, et al. Association between respiratory tract diseases and secondhand smoke exposure among never smoking flight attendants: A cross-sectional survey. *Environ Health.* 2007;6:28-36.
39. Chisti MJ, Tebruegge M, La Vincente S, et al. Pneumonia in severely malnourished children in developing countries - mortality risk, aetiology, and validity of WHO clinical signs: a systematic review. *Trop Med Int Health.* 2009;14:1173-89.

40. Sehgal V, Sethi GR, Sachdev HP, et al. Predictors of mortality in subjects hospitalized with acute lower respiratory tract infections. *Indian Pediatr.* 1997;34:213-19.
41. Tiewsoh K, Lodha R, Pandey RM, et al. Factors determining the outcome of children hospitalized with severe pneumonia. *BMC Pediatr.* 2009;9:15
42. Shah N, Ramankutty V, Premila PG, et al. Risk factors for severe pneumonia in children in south Kerala: A hospital-based case control study. *J Trop Pediatr.* 1994;40:201-6.
43. Mandell LA, Wunderink RG, Anzueto A, et al. Infectious Diseases Society of America/American Thoracic Society consensus guidelines on the management of community-acquired pneumonia in adults. *Clin Infect Dis.* 2007;44(2):S27-72.

World Clin Pulm Crit Care Med. 2019;6(1):12-26.

Etiological Diagnosis of Pneumonia

*Jyothi Edakalavan MD, Safreena M Nambipunnilath MD

Department of Pulmonary Medicine, Institute of Chest Diseases
Government Medical College, Kozhikode, Kerala, India

ABSTRACT

Pneumonia is diagnosed on the basis of signs and symptoms, supported by demonstrable radiographic infiltrate. However, certain situations warrant an etiological diagnosis which is mostly done by microbiological interventions. However, these tests are not always helpful, especially when the patient was put on an initial antibiotic therapy or when atypical organisms or rarer organisms cause the pneumonia. Even though there is a lack of consensus among experts about the composition of the diagnostic investigations for pneumonia, a well-chosen evaluation can support a diagnosis of pneumonia and identify a pathogen. Newer culture methods and molecular techniques have been evolved, which offer specific diagnosis in a shorter time frame. A well-chosen, individually tailored, evaluation can offer a lot of information to support the diagnosis of pneumonia.

INTRODUCTION

"I do not know any disease, which requires greater vigilance to detect in its first onset, than pneumonia in some of its varied forms and complications."

-Henry Duncalfe[1]

Making an early and accurate etiological diagnosis of pneumonia remains a challenge to this day. Despite the availability of sensitive diagnostic tests, the lack of a definitive microbiological diagnosis is often seen, especially in cases of community-acquired pneumonia (CAP). Atypical clinical presentations, infection

*Corresponding author
Email: drjyothie@yahoo.com

with drug-resistant or unusual organisms and unexpected complications make presumptive diagnosis and empirical treatment a risky option.

This article reviews various investigations in the etiological diagnosis of pneumonia giving special attention to include newer techniques like molecular methods.

MICROBIAL ETIOLOGY OF PNEUMONIA

The initial antimicrobial therapy is a key determinant in the successful treatment of pneumonia. Identification of the probable causative agent assists in choosing the appropriate antimicrobial therapy. The most practical approach to identify the etiological agent in pneumonia would be to begin with a classification into CAP, hospital-acquired pneumonia (HAP), and pneumonia in the immunocompromised host.

MICROBIAL ETIOLOGY OF COMMUNITY-ACQUIRED PNEUMONIA

The etiological diagnosis in CAP remains around 60% even with extensive investigations. In the outpatient setting, the most common pathogen causing CAP is *Streptococcus pneumoniae*. The introduction of pneumococcal vaccines and decreased rate of smoking has brought down the overall incidence of pneumococcal pneumonia. Atypical organisms like *Mycoplasma pneumoniae* and *Chlamydia pneumoniae*, followed by *Haemophilus influenzae*, are also common in the outpatient settings. *Streptococcus pneumoniae* affects older individuals while *Mycoplasma pneumoniae* affects previously healthy individuals younger than 50 years. Cyclic epidemics are known to occur with *Mycoplasma pneumoniae*.

In hospitalized patients, *Streptococcus pneumoniae* is the most common etiological agent. This organism is probably responsible for majority of the CAP cases with undetermined etiology. *Haemophilus influenzae, Mycoplasma pneumoniae, Chlamydia pneumoniae*, and *Legionella pneumophila* are also common in hospitalized patients.

Viral pneumonias are present in a high proportion of patients with CAP. The incidence of viral pneumonias can be as high as 80% during early childhood, but decreases to 5–20% in adults.[2] A systematic review and meta-analysis of 31 studies that evaluated viral infection in adult patients with CAP has identified influenza virus as the most common etiological agent, followed by rhinovirus, respiratory syncytial virus and corona virus.[3]

MICROBIAL ETIOLOGY OF HOSPITAL-ACQUIRED PNEUMONIA

Hospital-acquired pneumonia is defined as a pneumonia not incubating at the time of hospital admission and occurring 48 hours or more after admission. Early onset HAP is defined as a case that develops within the first 4 days of hospitalization. The common organisms implicated in early onset HAP are methicillin-sensitive *Staphylococcus aureus, Streptococcus pneumoniae, Haemophilus influenzae*, and anaerobes. Late onset HAP occurs after 5 days of hospitalization and tends to have a worse prognosis because of its association with multidrug resistant pathogens like methicillin-resistant *Staphylococcus aureus*, gram-negative bacilli like *Pseudomonas aeruginosa, Acinetobacter baumannii, Stenotrophomonas maltophilia*, and *Enterobacteriaceae* species. Gram-negative bacteria are implicated in 50–80% of the cases of HAP in an intensive care unit (ICU). Polymicrobial etiology is also frequent.[4]

CLINICAL PRESENTATION

Pneumonia can present with symptoms that may vary from mild to fatal in severity. The usual symptoms are fever, chills, cough, purulent sputum, pleuritic chest pain, and dyspnea. Atypical pneumonia or "walking pneumonia" has a more indolent course and are characterized by dry cough or cough with minimal expectoration. Relevant history can provide valuable clues regarding the etiologic agent of pneumonia (Table 1). Nonrespiratory manifestations may dominate the

Table 1: Etiological agents causing pneumonia

Type of pneumonia	Common organisms
Community-acquired pneumonia (CAP)	*Streptococcus pneumoniae, Haemophilus influenzae, Moraxella catarrhalis, Mycoplasma pneumoniae*, and respiratory viruses
Hospital-acquired pneumonia (HAP)	Early HAP: *Streptococcus pneumoniae, Haemophilus influenzae*, methicillin susceptible *Staphylococcus aureus*, antibiotic sensitive enteric Gram-negative bacilli Late HAP: Methicillin-resistant *Staphylococcus aureus, Pseudomonas aeruginosa, Klebsiella pneumoniae, Acinetobacter* spp., and *Legionella pneumophila*
Ventilator-associated pneumonia (VAP)	Early VAP: *Streptococcus pneumoniae, Haemophilus influenzae*, and methicillin susceptible *Staphylococcus aureus* Late VAP: *Pseudomonas aeruginosa, Enterobacter* spp., *Acinetobacter* spp., and methicillin-resistant *Staphylococcus aureus*
Pneumonia in the Immunocompromised	*Pneumocystis jirovecii, Toxoplasma gondii, Nocardia* spp., *Cytomegalovirus, Mycobacterium tuberculosis,* and *Aspergillus fumigatus*

clinical picture, especially in case of atypical pneumonias. Clinical features and history cannot reliably identify the specific etiology, or help in differentiating viral from bacterial infection.[5]

MICROBIOLOGICAL DIAGNOSIS OF PNEUMONIA

The role of microbiologic studies in determining the etiology of pneumonia is questionable, because of the lack of rapid, accurate, easy, and cost-effective methods, which can be obtained before starting treatment. Even in randomized controlled trials, the cause of CAP is determined in only 20–40% of cases.[6] However, in a study by Johansson et al. the microbial etiology of CAP could be identified in up to 67% of the patients by combining polymerase chain reaction (PCR) and conventional methods.[7]

Inadequate sputum sample, previous antibiotic therapy, and delay in processing the samples decrease the yield of Gram stain and culture. Pretreatment Gram stain and culture should be obtained only if a good quality specimen is available.[8] In CAP, sputum Gram staining and culture may be done in severe pneumonia and in patients admitted in intensive care units. The American Thoracic Society (ATS) pneumonia guidelines recommend sputum culture only if a drug-resistant pathogen, or an organism not covered by usual empiric therapy is suspected. Other indications put forth by Infectious Diseases Society of America (IDSA)/ATS guidelines include failure to respond to the initial empiric antibiotic, cavitary lesions in chest X-ray, history of alcohol abuse, underlying lung disease, a positive *Legionella* or pneumococcal urinary antigen. Sputum Gram stain and cultures are indicated for all patients with nosocomial pneumonia and ventilator-associated pneumonia as there is high-risk for the presence of multidrug resistant pathogens.[9]

The role of induced sputum at present is mainly for microbiological diagnosis in patients unable to produce sputum, especially children and immunosuppressed patients.[10] In a study by Lahti et al. involving 101 children, good quality sputum specimens were obtained from 76 children and a positive result was obtained in 90% of specimens.[11]

The other specimens from the lower respiratory tract include tracheal aspirate, bronchial washings, bronchoalveolar lavage (BAL), protected specimen brush (PSB) samples, bronchial biopsy, lung aspirates, and lung biopsy.

Gram Staining

Gram staining, originally devised, more than a century ago, is the standard method used for identifying microorganisms even today.[12] The commonly seen organisms in Gram stained smears include *S. pneumoniae* (gram-positive oval or lancet-shaped diplococci), *H. influenzae* (small pleomorphic gram-negative bacilli), and *M. catarrhalis* (gram-negative diplococci).[13] In nosocomial pneumonia, the infection is usually polymicrobial, and *S. aureus, P. aeruginosa*, *Enterobacter* spp., and *K. pneumoniae* are the commonly identified organisms.

Acid-fast Staining

The bacteriological examination of expectorated sputum for acid-fast bacilli (AFB) should be done in all patients with pneumonia, especially in developing countries. *M. tuberculosis* is typically a slightly curved or straight rod-shaped microbe (Figure 1). It is 1–4 mm in length and 0.3–0.6 mm in diameter.[13] *Mycobacterium tuberculosis* can be stained with carbolfuchsin [Ziehl-Neelsen (ZN) or Kinyoun] and fluorochrome stains. Auramine-Rhodamine staining is more sensitive than ZN staining, especially in paucibacillary cases, and the specificity is similar.[14,15]

Special Staining

Even though Gram staining and traditional culture methods are used routinely for the microbiological diagnosis of pneumonia, special staining methods are essential for the isolation of organisms in varying clinical situations. Potassium hydroxide (KOH) preparation of sputum for elastin fibers is a sensitive test for the diagnosis of necrotizing pneumonia.[16] In intubated patients, this can be done with bronchial washings. Potassium hydroxide preparation is also useful for identifying fungi in respiratory specimens.

Calcofluor white is a nonspecific fluorochrome stain that binds to fungi and *P. jirovecii*.[17] Modified Grocott-Gomori methenamine silver stain is used for staining *P. jirovecii* cysts, and Giemsa staining is used to stain the trophozoites.

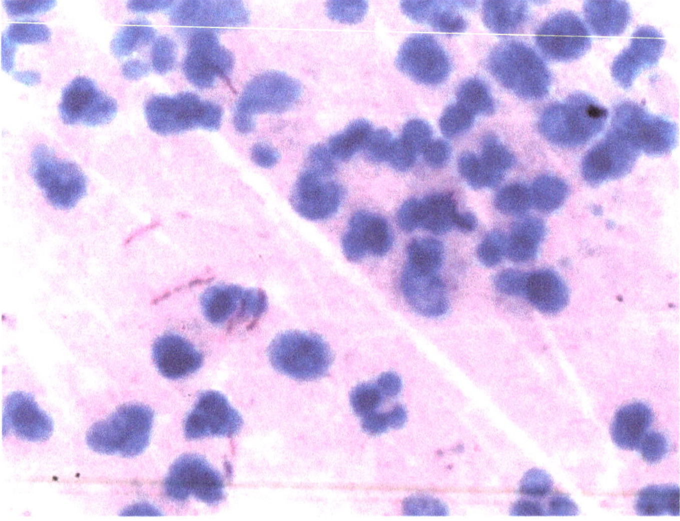

Figure 1: Sputum smear stained with Ziehl–Neelsen stain showing acid-fast bacilli.

The sensitivity for diagnosing *P. jirovecii* in expectorated sputum is less compared to bronchial washings and other invasive specimens.[18]

Sputum direct fluorescent antibody (DFA) is a rapid method for the diagnosis of respiratory pathogens. The sensitivity of DFA for Legionnaires' disease is less compared to *Legionella* urinary antigens, PCR, and culture. Direct fluorescent antibody tests are also available for detecting *P. jirovecii* and it was found that there was little difference between expectorated and induced sputum, when DFA was used for the diagnosis of *Pneumocystis jirovecii* pneumonia.[19]

Culture Methods

Routine culture methods for microbiological diagnosis are slow, the sensitivity is low, and the result may be influenced by prior antibiotic therapy. It is recommended that before starting the patient on empiric therapy, a sputum sample should be sent for culture and sensitivity. In a study by Rello et al. positive microbiological test resulted in treatment modification in 41.6% of patients, including 5% of patients in whom the initial antimicrobials were ineffective against the isolated organism.[20] A positive microbiological diagnosis helps in de-escalation of therapy, minimizes the emergence of drug resistance and reduces the treatment cost.[21]

Traditionally, sputum culture is done on the following media—blood agar, chocolate agar, and MacConkey agar. *Legionella* grows on selective media (Buffered Charcoal Yeast Extract) after 48 hours incubation at 37°C in aerobic conditions.

If fungal infection is suspected, sputum should be cultured on Sabouraud's agar. For the detection of *M. tuberculosis*, both conventional and rapid culture methods are available. Conventional culture media like Lowenstein-Jensen medium takes up to 6 weeks for obtaining a positive culture (Figure 2). The available rapid culture

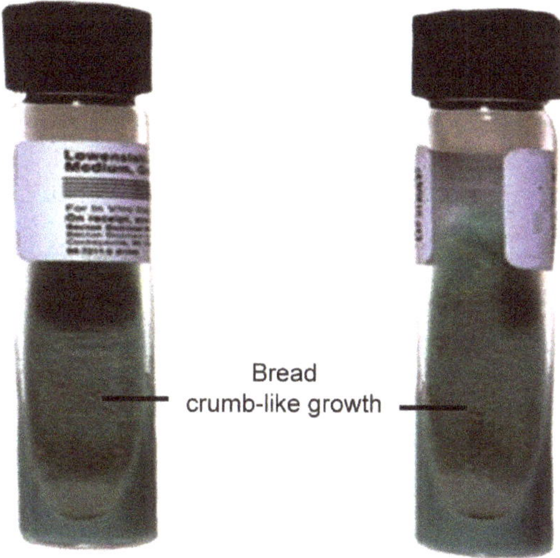

Figure 2: *Mycobacterum tuberculosis* grown in Lowenstein-Jensen medium.

methods for *M. tuberculosis* are BACTEC culture medium, mycobacterial growth indicator tube, septi-check AFB, and MB/BacT system.

Blood Culture

Blood cultures are used to identify the organism and to guide the treatment. The IDSA and ATS guidelines recommend two blood samples for patients admitted to the hospital with pneumonia. The overall yield of blood culture is below 20%. In a study by Campbell et al., the rate of modification of treatment based on blood culture reports was only 1.97%.[22] In another study by Abe et al., a positive blood culture was obtained in 3.7% and resulted in change of antibiotics in only 2.4% of patients.[23] In a study by Waterer et al., the yield of positive blood culture increased with pneumonia severity index (PSI) grade, increasing to 26.7% in PSI grade V and resulted in a change in antibiotic treatment in 20% of patients.[24] Therefore, to reduce expenditure and to preserve resources, it is recommended to restrict blood culture to high-risk patients.

Urinary Antigen

Immunochromatographic tests in urine are rapid and noninvasive tests to identify *Legionella* and pneumococci. The results are not modified by prior antibiotic treatment. Studies in adults showed a sensitivity of 70% and specificity of 89.7% for the diagnosis of pneumococcal pneumonia.[25,26] The disadvantage of urinary antigen is the cost and the lack of an organism isolated for drug susceptibility testing. The test will be positive for several weeks to months after the illness.

Legionella urinary antigen is 76% sensitive and more than 90% specific for *L. pneumophila* serogroup-1.[27] *Legionella* urinary antigen detection is not recommended as a routine investigation for hospitalized patients with CAP, as narrowing antibiotic spectrum based on the results has a higher risk of clinical relapse.[28]

Nucleic Acid Amplification Test

Polymerase chain reaction detects microbial nucleic acid from cultured sample or direct respiratory specimen (Table 2). It helps in pathogen-directed therapy at the time of starting initial antibiotics.

Multiplex PCR is a variant of PCR which enables simultaneous amplification of many targets in one reaction by using more than one pair of primers so that multiple respiratory pathogens can be identified in a single test. In a study by Templeton et al., on 358 respiratory samples over 1 year period, respiratory viruses were detected by viral culture in 67 (19%) samples and by multiplex PCR in

Table 2: Comparative Outcome of Polymerase Chain Reaction and Culture in Pneumonia

Study	Polymerase chain reaction	Culture
Resti et al.[31]	45 of 292 (15.4%)	11 of 292 (3.8%)
Deng et al.[32]		
S. pneumoniae	32 of 176 (18.1%)	7 of 176 (4%)
H. influenzae	29 of 176 (16.4%)	23 of 176 (13%)
Menéndez et al.[33] (*S. pneumoniae*-blood)	41 of 184 (22.2%)	7 of 184 (3.8%)
Guclu et al.[34]	67 of 107 (62.6%)	33 of 107 (31%)
Mervat Gamal Eldin (endotracheal aspirate)	19 of 25 (76%)	6 of 25 (24%)
Mansour (Nosocomial pneumonia- blood)	17 of 25 (68%)	2 of 25 (8%)
Templeton et al.[29]	87 of 358 (24%)	67 of 358 (19%)

87 (24%) samples, showing that PCR was sensitive in detecting respiratory virus than culture.[29]

Real time-PCR combines the standard PCR method with fluorescent probe detection of the amplified product.[30] Since, the amplified product detection is also done simultaneously, results can be obtained very fast so that specific treatment decisions can be done based on the results.

Real time-PCR can also be used to detect the DNA quantitatively and thus, will be able to differentiate between colonization and infection. Induced sputum was obtained from the patients, and it was evaluated for the presence of *P. jirovecii* DNA using conventional PCR and real-time PCR. Conventional PCR had a high false-positive rate of 46.4% as it was positive in patients with colonization, also.[35] Concentration of DNA detected by real time PCR was significantly higher in pneumocystis patients than in colonizers.

There are no United States Food and Drug Administration (FDA) approved PCR tests for *S. pneumoniae*. For the diagnosis of *M. pneumoniae*, the sensitivity of PCR is less compared to serology.[36] Polymerase chain reaction for the diagnosis of tuberculosis is most useful in patients with positive acid-fast smears. A negative PCR in a smear negative patient will not rule out tuberculosis. Many novel multiplex real time PCR have been developed for the differentiation of *M. tuberculosis* complex strains.[37,38]

The area where PCR has greatest impact on pathogen identification in pneumonia is in the identification of respiratory viruses. Reverse transcriptase (RT-PCR) is used to detect RNA viruses. This was extremely useful in the management of hantavirus epidemics in New Mexico, severe acute respiratory syndrome (SARS) epidemic in Asia, the H1N1 epidemic of 2009, and the Middle East respiratory syndrome (MERS) corona virus epidemic of Saudi Arabia.[39]

The major problem with PCR assay is the risk of false-positive results. This can result from contamination by exogenous material or by detection of colonizing organisms as a result of the extreme sensitivity of PCR assay.

Serology

Serologic tests may be useful to establish the cause of pneumonia when the causative agents are difficult to isolate. A four-fold or greater rise in titer between acute and convalescent sera is required for the diagnosis, so it is not useful in the initial antibiotic selection for treatment. The antibodies may persist for months or years after an initial *Legionella* infection. Thus, a single titer of 1:256 or higher may reflect a prior *Legionella* infection. Serologic tests may be useful for the epidemiologic al diagnosis. The commonly diagnosed infections by serology are *L. pneumophila, C. psittaci, M. pneumoniae, C. burnetii*, and *F. tularensis.* Serologic tests may also be useful in the retrospective diagnosis of infections due to influenza A and B, respiratory syncytial virus, adenovirus, and parainfluenza virus. Several serologic assays have been developed for detection of antibodies in MERS. The Centers for Disease Control and Prevention has developed a two phase serologic testing for surveillance and not for diagnostic purpose. The enzyme-linked immunosorbent assay is done as a screening test and if this is found to be positive, an indirect immunofluorescence or microneutralization assay is done for confirmation.[39]

Levels of interleukin (IL)-1b and IL-8 in BAL fluid are the strongest markers for accurately identifying ventilator-associated pneumonia (VAP). Based on this, it is possible to reduce unnecessary antibiotic use in suspected VAP patients, but this requires further validation in larger populations.[40] Mid-regional proatrial natriuretic peptide and C-terminal proatrial vasopressin estimation are the new and emerging tools for the prediction of short-term and long-term risk stratification of patients with CAP.[41]

INVASIVE DIAGNOSTIC PROCEDURES

Invasive diagnostic procedures are advised in pneumonia in the following situations:

- Slowly resolving or nonresolving pneumonia
- Patients having life-threatening complications
- Pneumonia in immunocompromised host
- HAP or VAP.

Thoracentesis

Parapneumonic effusions (PPEs) are seen in more than 40% of patients with bacterial pneumonia. It is seen in up to 60% of patients with pneumococcal pneumonia. Small pleural effusions are seen in viral and *Mycoplasma pneumoniae* in up to 20% of patients. *S. aureus* is the commonly isolated organism in empyema thoracic in postsurgical patients.[42] If there is associated pleural effusion or empyema, every effort should be taken to retrieve adequate quantity of fluid for establishing an etiological diagnosis. Diagnostic thoracentesis can aid in the diagnosis and treatment plan for almost all pleural effusions. All PPEs having a thickness of more than 10 mm on the lateral decubitus X-ray, ultrasound, or computed tomography (CT) scan should be subjected for sampling.[43]

Transthoracic Needle Aspiration

Transthoracic needle aspiration (TNA) is an easy procedure to carry out with very few complications and well tolerated by most of the patients. In a study by Hernes et al., a definite etiology of CAP was obtained in 60% of patients with TNA.[44]

Bronchoscopic Techniques

Bronchoscopic procedure is used for collecting uncontaminated specimens for quantitative or qualitative cultures. Quantitative cultures have been demonstrated to have good diagnostic utility for the presence of pneumonia, especially in patients with a low or equivocal clinical suspicion of infection.[45] Consistent recovery of potential pathogens with invasive techniques can identify patients at high-risk of mortality.[46] To differentiate between infection and colonization, the diagnostic threshold varies with the technique used. Bronchoscopic BAL uses a diagnostic threshold of 104 or 105 cfu/mL. Protected specimen brush samples require a diagnostic threshold of 103 cfu/mL or more. Protected specimen brush is more specific than sensitive for diagnosing pneumonia.[47,48]

Nonbronchoscopic Technique

The nonbronchoscopic technique involves passage of a catheter through the endotracheal tube, and then it is advanced and wedged into the bronchus. Samples are taken with a catheter containing a brush (blind PSB),[49] or by aspiration of secretions through a distally wedged catheter. Bronchoalveolar lavage may be performed by using a balloon-tipped catheter with the balloon inflated after the catheter has been advanced to the wedged position (protected BAL) also called nonbronchoscopic BAL or mini BAL. The yield of bronchoscopic and nonbronchoscopic technique for obtaining quantitative cultures of lower respiratory specimens is comparable.[50]

Lung Biopsy

In very severe cases of pneumonia or when the diagnosis is not clear, particularly in patients with a damaged immune system, a lung biopsy may be required. This can be done by bronchoscopic biopsy, needle aspiration, open lung biopsy, or video-assisted thoracoscopic biopsy. Open lung biopsy through a very limited anterior thoracotomy is employed in the diagnosis of *Pneumocystis jirovecii* pneumonia. Gaensler et al.[51] demonstrated the high yield of positive diagnoses by this procedure in diffuse pneumonic processes. Routine permanent section stains and cultures of lung tissue for bacteria and fungi. Acid-fast bacilli should also be performed.

Role of Biomarkers in Diagnosis of Pneumonia

The differentiation of bacterial pneumonia from viral and other noninfectious etiology is important in the emergency setting. Biomarkers like C-reactive protein and procalcitonin have been widely studied in pneumonia. C-reactive protein is a sensitive inflammatory biomarker, but has low specificity in the diagnosis of pneumonias.[52] The most useful biomarker in pneumonia appears to be procalcitonin, the hormone precursor of calcitonin. The conversion of procalcitonin to calcitonin is inhibited by bacterial endotoxins and cytokines. Procalcitonin concentrations in the serum of healthy subjects are undetectable or low, generally less than 0.1 ng/mL. A procalcitonin level of 0.25 ng/mL or higher in the setting of pneumonia predicts a bacterial infection as the likely cause.[53] Procalcitonin levels more than 2 ng/mL in CAP was associated with an increased incidence of bacteremia, septic shock, multiorgan failure, and mortality.[54] A Cochrane meta-analysis found that antibiotic use based on procalcitonin values was associated with reduction in antibiotic use, without increase in mortality or treatment failure.[55] However, the 2016 IDSA guideline for HAP recommends that the decision to start on antibiotics should be based on clinical criteria alone, rather than using serum procalcitonin plus clinical criteria.[9]

CONCLUSION

Community-acquired pneumonia is diagnosed on the basis of symptoms and signs and a radiographic abnormality. However, certain situations warrant an etiological diagnosis, which is mostly by microbiological intervention. However, these tests are not always helpful, especially when the patient is put on an initial antibiotic therapy or when atypical organisms or rarer organisms cause pneumonia. Newer culture methods and molecular technique have been evolved, which offer specific diagnosis in a shorter time frame. A well-chosen, individually tailored evaluation can offer information to support the diagnosis of pneumonia.

Editor's Comment

Diagnosis of pneumonia has mainly been on the basis of clinical and radiological picture. It has been felt that the utility of tests to establish the etiology of pneumonia is much below the expectations. This is mainly because the tests like Gram staining are not very specific and culture takes time. The treatment of community-acquired pneumonia has, therefore, been mainly empirical. In patients with severe community-acquired pneumonia and hospital-acquired pneumonia, there has been more aggressive approach to make an etiological diagnosis and often more invasive tests are employed. With advances in technology, a number of rapid tests have emerged for the early diagnosis of pneumonia. Molecular tests like polymerase chain reaction have a high sensitivity and specificity. Urinary antigen tests for pneumococci and legionella are now available. Rapid diagnostic tests for viral pneumonia have revolutionized the diagnosis of pneumonia due to most of the viral pathogens. In the future one hopes to have rapid, point of care, and cost effective methods for the detection of etiological agents causing pneumonia. In this article, the authors elaborated most of the diagnostic methods available to identify the etiology in pneumonia.

Ravindran Chetambath

REFERENCES

1. Duncalfe H. On some of the varieties and complications of pneumonia. *BMJ.* 1857:67.
2. Blasi F, Aliberti S, Pappalettera M, et al. 100 years of respiratory medicine: Pneumonia. *Respir Med.* 2007;101:875-81.
3. Burk M, El-Kersh K, Saad M, et al. Viral infection in community-acquired pneumonia: A systematic review and meta-analysis. *Eur Respir Rev.* 2016;25:178-88.
4. Cilloniz C, Martin-Loeches I, Gaarcia-Vidal C, et al. Microbial etiology of pneumonia: Epidemiology, diagnosis and resistance patterns. *Int J Mol Sci.* 2016;17:2120.
5. Brar NK, Niederman MS. Management of community-acquired pneumonia: A review and update. *Ther Adv Respir Dis.* 2011;5(1):61-78.
6. Fine MJ, Stone RA, Singer DE, et al. Processes and outcomes of care for patients with community-acquired pneumonia: Results from the Pneumonia Patient Outcomes Research Team cohort study. *Arch Intern Med.* 1999;159:970-80.

7. Johansson N, Kalin M, Tiveljung-Lindell A, et al. Etiology of community-acquired pneumonia: Increased microbiological yield with new diagnostic methods. *Clin Infect Dis.* 2010;50:202-9.
8. Mandell LA, Wunderink RG, Bartlett JG, et al. Infectious Diseases Society of America; American Thoracic Society. Infectious Diseases Society of America/American Thoracic Society consensus guidelines on management of community-acquired pneumonia in adults. *Clin Infect Dis.* 2007;44:S27-72.
9. Kalil AC, Metersky ML, Klompas M. Management of adults with hospital-acquired and ventilator-associated pneumonia: 2016 clinical practice guidelines by the Infectious Diseases Society of America and the American Thoracic Society. *Clin Infect Dis.* 2016:63.
10. da Silva RM, Teixeira PJ, Moreira Jda S. The clinical utility of induced sputum for the diagnosis of bacterial community-acquired pneumonia in HIV infected patients: A prospective cross-sectional study. *Braz J Infect Dis.* 2006;10:89-93.
11. Lahti E, Peltola V, Waris M, et al. Induced sputum in the diagnosis of childhood community-acquired pneumonia. *Thorax.* 2009;64:252-57.
12. Moyes RB, Reynolds J, Breakwell DP. Differential staining of bacteria: Gram stain. *Curr Protoc Microbiol.* 2009; Appendix 3: Appendix 3C.
13. Michael DI. Biology and laboratory diagnosis of tuberculosis: A clinicians' guide to tuberculosis. Lippincott Williams & Wilkins. 2000. pp. 22.
14. Ba F, Rieder HL. A comparison of fluorescence microscopy with the Ziehl-Neelsen technique in the examination of sputum for acid-fast bacilli. *Int J Tuberc Lun Dis.* 1999;3:1101-105.
15. Steingart KR, Henry M, Ng V, et al. Fluorescence versus conventional sputum smear microscopy for tuberculosis: A systematic review. *Lancet Infect Dis.* 2006;6:570-81.
16. Shlaes DM, Lederman MM, Chmielewski R, et al. Sputum elastin fibers and the diagnosis of necrotizing pneumonia. *Chest.* 1984;85:763-66.
17. Kim YK, Parulekar S, Yu PK, et al. Evaluation of calcofluor white stain for detection of Pneumocystis carinii. *Diagn Microbiol Infect Dis.* 1990;13:307-10.
18. Aslanzadeh J, Stelmach PS. Detection of Pneumocystis carinii with direct fluorescence antibody and calcofluor white stain. *Infection.* 1996;24:248-50.
19. Metersky ML, Aslenzadeh J, Stelmach P. A comparison of induced and expectorated sputum in the diagnosis of Pneumocystis carinii pneumonia. *Chest.* 1998;113:1555-59.
20. Rello J, Bodi M, Mariscal D, et al. Microbiological testing and outcome of patients with severe community-acquired pneumonia. *Chest.* 2003;123:174-80.
21. Dellit TH, Owens RC, McGowan JE, et al. Infectious Diseases Society of America and the Society for Healthcare Epidemiology of America guidelines for developing an institutional program to enhance antimicrobial stewardship. *Clin Infect Dis.* 2007;44:159-77.
22. Campbell SG, Marrie TJ, Anstey R, et al. The contribution of blood cultures to the clinical management of adult patients admitted to the hospital with community-acquired pneumonia: A prospective observational study. *Chest.* 2003;123:1142-50.
23. Abe T, Tokuda Y, Ishimatsu S, et al. Usefulness of initial blood cultures in patients admitted with pneumonia from an emergency department in Japan. *J Infect Chemother.* 2009;15:180-86.
24. Waterer GW, Wunderink RG. The influence of the severity of community-acquired pneumonia on the usefulness of blood culture. *Respir Med.* 2001;95:78-82.
25. Gutiérrez F, Masiá M, Rodríguez JC, et al. Evaluation of the immunochromatographic Binax NOW assay for detection of Streptococcus pneumoniae urinary antigen in a prospective study of community-acquired pneumonia in Spain. *Clinical Inf Dis.* 2003;36:286-92.
26. Smith MD, Sheppard CL, Hogan A, et al. Diagnosis of Streptococcus pneumoniae infections in adults with bacteremia and community-acquired pneumonia: Clinical comparison of pneumococcal PCR and urinary antigen detection. *J Clin Microbiol.* 2009;47:1046-69.
27. Yu VL, Stout JE. Rapid diagnostic testing for community-acquired pneumonia: Can innovative technology for clinical microbiology be exploited? *Chest.* 2009;136:1618-21.

28. Falguera M, Ruiz-González A, Schoenenberger JA, et al. Prospective, randomised study to compare empirical treatment versus targeted treatment on the basis of the urine antigen results in hospitalized patients with community-acquired pneumonia. *Thorax.* 2010;65:101-106.
29. Templeton KE, Scheltinga SA, Beersma MF, et al. Rapid and sensitive method using multiplex real-time PCR for diagnosis of infections by influenza A and influenza B viruses, respiratory syncytial virus, and parainfluenza viruses 1, 2, 3, and 4. *J Clin Microbiol.* 2004;42:1564-69.
30. Espy MJ, Uhl JR, Sloan LM, et al. Real-time PCR in clinical microbiology: Applications for routine laboratory testing. *Clin Microbiol Rev.* 2006;19:165-56.
31. Resti M, Moriondo M, Cortimiglia M, et al. Community-acquired bacteremic pneumococcal pneumonia in children: Diagnosis and serotyping by real-time polymerase chain reaction using blood samples. *Clin Infect Dis.* 2010;51:1042-49.
32. Deng J, Zheng Y, Zhao R, et al. Culture versus polymerase chain reaction for the etiologic diagnosis of community-acquired pneumonia in antibiotic-pretreated pediatric patients. *Pediatr Infect Dis J.* 2009;28:53-55.
33. Menéndez R, Córdoba C, de La Cuadra P, et al. Value of the polymerase chain reaction assay in noninvasive respiratory samples for diagnosis of community-acquired pneumonia. *Am J Respir Crit Care Med.* 1999;159:1868-73.
34. Guclu AU, Baysallar M, Gozen AG, et al. Polymerase chain reaction vs. conventional culture in detection of bacterial pneumonia agents. *Ann Microbiol.* 2005;55:313-16.
35. Fujisawa T, Suda T, Matsuda H, et al. Real-time PCR is more specific than conventional PCR for induced sputum diagnosis of Pneumocystis pneumonia in immunocompromised patients without HIV infection. *Respirology.* 2009;14:203-9.
36. Martínez MA, Ruiz M, Zunino E, et al. Detection of Mycoplasma pneumoniae in adult community-acquired pneumonia by PCR and serology. *J Med Microbiol.* 2008;57:1491-95.
37. Halse TA, Escuyer VE, Musser KA. Evaluation of a single tube multiplexes real-time PCR for differentiation of members of the Mycobacterium tuberculosis complex in clinical specimens. *J Clin Microbiol.* 2011;49: 2562-67.
38. Reddington K, O'Grady J, Dorai-Raj S, et al. Novel multiplex real-time PCR diagnostic assay for identification and differentiation of Mycobacterium tuberculosis, Mycobacterium canettii, and Mycobacterium tuberculosis complex strains. *J Clin Microbiol.* 2011;49:651-57.
39. Centres for disease control and prevention. CDC Laboratory Testing for Middle East Respiratory Syndrome Coronavirus (MERS-CoV). 2014. [Accessed on 25 Jun 2017] Available from: www.cdc.gov/coronavirus/mers/lab/lab-testing.html.
40. Conway Morris A, Kefala K, Wilkinson TS, et al. Diagnostic importance of pulmonary interleukin-1b and interleukin-8 in ventilator-associated pneumonia. *Thorax.* 2010;65:201-207.
41. Krüger S, Ewig S, Kunde J, et al. Pro-atrial natriuretic peptide and provasopressin for predicting short-term and long-term survival in community-acquired pneumonia: Results from the German Competence Network CAPNETZ. *Thorax.* 2010;65:208-14.
42. Grijalva CG, Zhu Y, Nuorti JP, et al. Emergence of parapneumonic empyema in the USA. *Thorax.* 2011;66: 663-68.
43. Rahman NM, Chapman SJ, Davies RJ. The approach to the patient with a parapneumonic effusion. *Clin Chest Med.* 2008;27:253-66.
44. Hernes SS, Hagen E, Tofteland S, et al. Transthoracic fine-needle aspiration in the aetiological diagnosis of community acquired pneumonia. *Clin Microbiol Infect.* 2010;16(7):909-11.
45. Heyland DK, Cook DJ, Marshall J, et al. The clinical utility of invasive diagnostic techniques in the setting of ventilator-associated pneumonia. Canadian Critical Care Trials Group. *Chest.* 1999;115:1076-84.
46. Rello J, Gallego M, Mariscal D, et al. The value of routine microbial investigation in ventilator associated pneumonia. *Am J Respir Crit Care Med.* 1997;156:196-200.
47. Marquette CH, Herengt F, Mathieu D, et al. Diagnosis of pneumonia in mechanically ventilated patients. Repeatability of the protected specimen brush. *Am Rev Respir Dis.* 1993;147:211-14.

48. Torres A, El-Ebiary M. Bronchoscopic BAL in the diagnosis of ventilator-associated pneumonia. *Chest.* 2000;117:198S-202S.
49. Torres A, de la Bellacasa JP, Rodriguez-Roisin R, et al. Diagnostic value of telescoping plugged catheters in mechanically ventilated patients with bacterial pneumonia using the Metras catheter. *Am Rev Respir Dis.* 1988;138:117-20.
50. Torres A, Ewig S. Diagnosing ventilator-associated pneumonia. *N Engl J Med.* 2004;350:433-35.
51. Gaensler EA, Moister VB, Hamm J. Open-lung biopsy in diffuse pulmonary disease. *N Engl J Med.* 1964;270:1319-31.
52. Almirall J, Bolibar I, Toran P, et al. Contribution of C-reactive protein to the diagnosis and assessment of severity of community acquired pneumonia. *Chest.* 2004;125:1335-42.
53. Smi NJ, Samson DJ, Galaydick JL, et al. Procalcitonin guided antibiotic therapy: A systematic review and meta-analysis. *J Hosp Med.* 2013;8:530-40.
54. Boussekey N, Leroy O, Georges H, et al. Diagnostic and prognostic values of admission procalcitonin levels in community-acquired pneumonia in an intensive care unit. *Infection.* 2005;33(4):257–63.
55. Schuetz P, Müller B, Christ-Crain M, et al. Procalcitonin to initiate or discontinue antibiotics in acute respiratory tract infections. *Cochrane Database Syst Rev.* 2017;10:CD007498.

World Clin Pulm Crit Care Med. 2019;6(1):27-48.

Role of Imaging in Respiratory Infections

[1]Bhavin Dalal MD DNB MNAMS FCCP, [2]Ishani Dalal MD DMRD,
[3,*]Korembeth P Ravikrishnan FRCP FACP FCCP

[1,3]Department of Internal Medicine, Division of Pulmonary and Critical Care, William Beaumont Hospital
Oakland University School of Medicine, Royal Oak, Michigan, USA
[2]Department of Radiology and Nuclear Medicine, Henry Ford Health System
Detroit, Michigan, USA

ABSTRACT

Radiographic imaging is an early diagnostic study performed in patients with pneumonia. There have been great advances in the imaging procedures since the original use of chest radiograph in the diagnosis of pneumonia. A chest radiograph is the gold standard for the initial diagnosis of pneumonia. Consensus guidelines of American Thoracic Society (ATS) and the Infectious Disease Society of North America (IDSA) require a radiograph for the diagnosis of pneumonia. Pneumonia and its complications can be identified by several imaging techniques like plain chest radiograph, computerized tomographic (CT) scan, ultrasound of lung and the findings and signs in these images help the radiologists and clinicians every day in the diagnosis and management of pneumonia.

INTRODUCTION

This article is a comprehensive review of the role of imaging methods in the evaluation of patients with infectious pneumonia. Ever since the original and classic description of radiographic findings of air-bronchogram and consolidation of lobar pneumonia by Dr Benjamin Felson and Dr Felix Fleischner, close to a century ago there has been tremendous advancements in the field of radiology in the detection of pneumonia and its complications.[1,2] Radiological patterns are determined by the pathological and the structural changes in the lung parenchyma, the airways and the thoracic cavity due to the infection and the inflammatory

*Corresponding author
Email: k.ravikrishnan@beaumont.edu

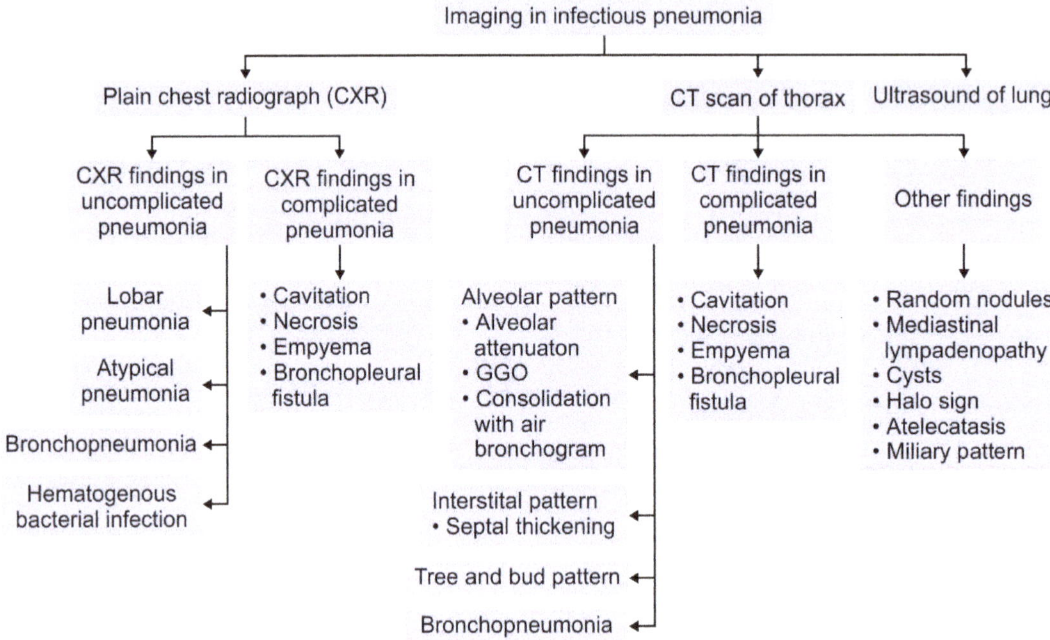

CXR, chest X-ray; CT, computed tomography; GGO, ground-glass opacity.

Figure 1: Summary of radiological findings in patients with infectious pneumonia.

response secondary to infection. This article describes the findings of infectious pneumonia in plain chest radiograph, computed tomography (CT) scan, and ultrasound as outlined in figure 1.

CHEST RADIOGRAPHS

A chest radiograph is the gold standard for the initial diagnosis of pneumonia. Consensus guidelines of the American Thoracic Society (ATS) and the Infectious disease society of North America (IDSA) require a radiograph for the diagnosis of pneumonia.[3] Opacities in the chest radiographs are characteristic findings in respiratory infections and the diagnosis of pneumonia rests on this finding seen in the initial radiograph. Early during pulmonary infection, the inflammation in the lung parenchyma leads to alveolar and interstitial pattern to varying extent. Pathological classification helps the clinicians to define radiographic findings and signs of pneumonia.[4] In cases of pneumonia, diagnostic accuracy of the initial chest radiograph approaches to 80–90%.[5,6] In addition to helping with the early diagnosis of pneumonia, chest radiograph helps to stratify the severity of pneumonia. Involvement of multiple lobes, associated pleural involvement and evidence of other complications help to define severity of community-acquired pneumonia.[7]

Chest X-ray Scan Findings in Uncomplicated Pneumonia

In an uncomplicated pneumonia, four distinct radiographic patterns have been described which include: (i) lobar pneumonia, (ii) atypical pneumonia, (iii) bronchopneumonia, (iv) hematogenous bacterial infection.

Lobar Pneumonia

A dense homogenous opacification of a segment or a lobe with intact air-filled airways (air-bronchogram) are pathognomonic of pneumonia, often by a bacterial organism.[8] Air-bronchogram is a characteristic radiographic finding of consolidation and can be clinically correlated with the finding of bronchial breath sounds on auscultation. Airways are spared in this homogenous opacification and there is no volume loss as in the case of atelectasis.[8,9] This characteristic presentation of streptococcal pneumonia (*S. pneumoniae*) often with single lobe involvement has earned the name "lobar pneumonia," which is the most common cause of community-acquired pneumonia (Figure 2). The tissue plains are well respected in uncomplicated pneumonia. Radiographic findings of consolidation can coexist with findings of pleural effusion in up to 10% of cases of *S. pneumoniae*. Gram-negative infections usually produce multilobar and diffuse parenchymal abnormalities. At times, involvement of a single lobe with increase in the exudative volume causes a lobar pneumonia pattern with a "bulging fissure sign" as in the case of *Klebsiella* pneumonia and other virulent gram-negative pneumonias (Figure 3).

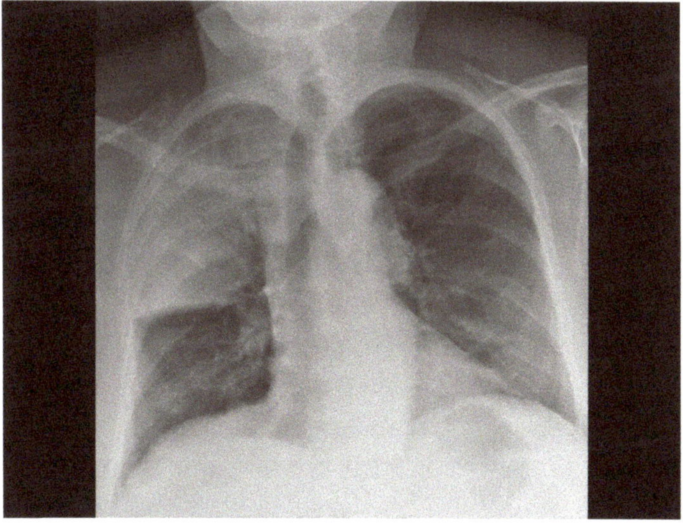

Figure 2: The chest X-ray showing opacification of right upper lobe sharply limited by minor fissure due to airspace consolidation with air-bronchogram most likely due to pneumococcal pneumonia.

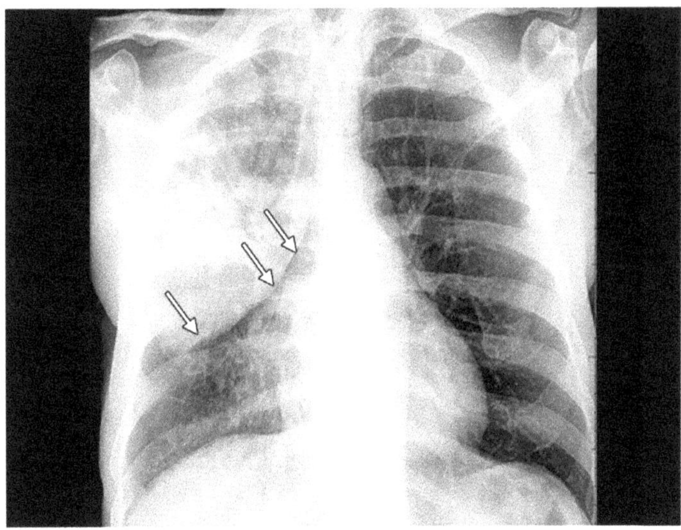

Figure 3: Dense consolidation of right upper lobe with air-bronchogram. Arrows point toward bulging fissure sign.

Atypical Pneumonia/Interstitial Pneumonia

Clinicians and radiologists have noted an atypical pattern of alveolar and interstitial involvement ever since the use of chest radiographs as a diagnostic modality. Poorly marginated fluffy alveolar involvement with linear markings suggestive of an interstitial pattern was noted quite dissimilar to the classic lobar pneumonia. This multilobar pattern was referred to as atypical pneumonia and was often caused by an atypical microbe like *Mycoplasma pneumoniae* (Figure 4). In atypical pneumonia, radiographic findings usually do not correlate the clinical state which is known as clinico-radiological dissociation. Radiological abnormalities can be present beyond the clinical resolution of pneumonia. Over the years this pattern has been described in association with other infections like chlamydia, psittacosis, Q-fever, and viral pneumonia and it has become very clear that there is nothing atypical about atypical pneumonia pattern. Diffuse and progressive involvement of lung parenchyma with early evidence of acute lung injury is noted in emerging viral infection and epidemics as in cases of H1N1 infections.[10,11] Though there are no specific patterns for viral pneumonia, bilateral, extensive, and dense consolidative pattern are noted as in case of varicella pneumonia. Varicella pneumonia also has been known to cause an acute interstitial pneumonia in adults. If interstitial pattern is present in immunocompetent host, it is often due to *Mycoplasma*, *Chlamydia* (TWAR), *Haemophilus influenzae*, *Legionella*, or viral pathogens.[9] Acute influenza pneumonia presents as an acute interstitial pneumonia and can rapidly progress to acute respiratory distress syndrome (ARDS) with diffuse alveolar damage indistinguishable from noninfectious causes of diffuse alveolar damage.[8] A self-limiting influenza like acute interstitial presentation has been reported with

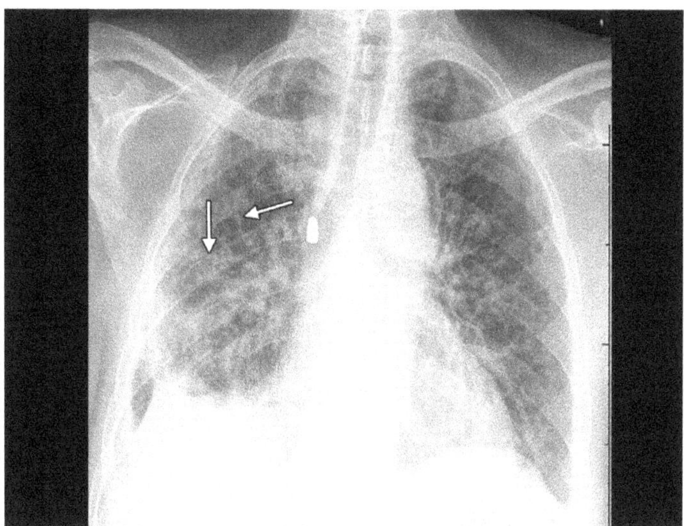

Figure 4: Multilobar diffuse interstitial pneumonia can be seen with atypical infectious causes like *Mycoplasma pneumoniae*, viral pneumonia. Of note, this pattern can be seen with noninfectious conditions as well (arrows show reticular markings).

overwhelming exposure to histoplasmosis, blastomycosis, and coccidioidomycosis even in an immunocompetent host. In immunocompromised hosts, any infection can be overwhelming and a diffuse bilateral acute interstitial pattern can be seen in cases of *Pneumocystis jirovecii* pneumonia (PJP), *cytomegalovirus* (CMV), tuberculosis (TB), cryptococcosis, nocardiosis, and nontuberculous mycobacteria. An acute organizing pneumonia without any findings and evidence of architectural distortions can be seen in many noninfectious interstitial pneumonia and can be indistinguishable. Radiographic findings are often disproportionate to clinical findings and the delay in resolution of the pattern should alert the clinicians of the possibility of noninfectious causes.[12]

Bronchopneumonia

The radiographic findings with extensive parenchymal involvement are a feature of more virulent gram-positive and gram-negative organisms. Tissue plains are not well respected and the radiographic appearance is characterized by ill-defined nodular opacities with confluent shadows and multilobar involvement (Figure 5). Infiltrates go beyond the fissures involving multiple segments and lobes. Early tissue necrosis and caseation leads to cavity formation and pleural involvement, and complex pleural effusions are common. Staphylococcal pneumonia appears as bronchopneumonia with bilateral fluffy nodular involvement and formation of early pneumatoceles occurring as clear airspaces or fluid filled cavities. This pattern should be recognized early in the cases of community-acquired methicillin-

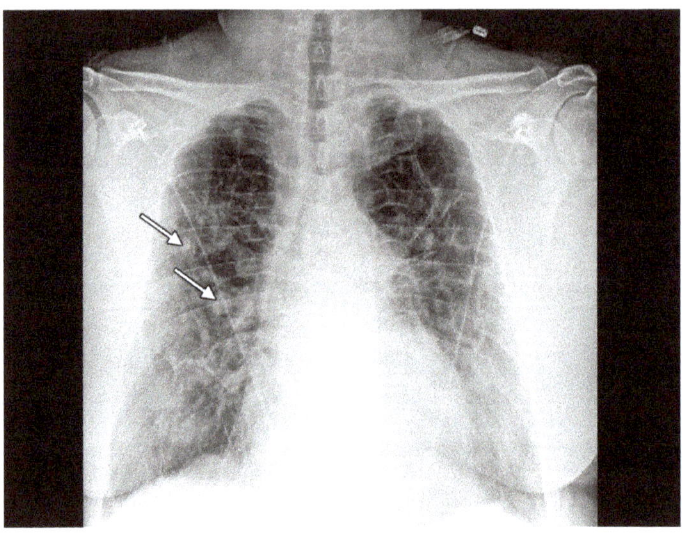

Figure 5: Bronchopneumonia: Ill-defined patchy nodular opacities with confluent shadows and multi lobar involvement (arrows point toward nodular opacities).

resistant *Staphylococcus aureus* (MRSA) infection because of the high mortality associated with delay in the diagnosis. Gram-negative infections like *Escherichia coli, Pseudomonas* spp., and other enteric gram-negative bacteria present with extensive bilateral bronchopneumonia pattern and are usually causative organisms in hospital-acquired pneumonia.

Hematogenous Bacterial Infection

Bilateral pneumonia associated with bacteremia is a common presentation of MRSA especially among intravenous drug addicts. Septic pulmonary infarcts are often characterized by diffuse nodular fluffy opacities often with cavities seen bilaterally particularly in vascular distribution (Figure 6).

Chest X-ray Finding in Complicated Pneumonia

Infectious pneumonia can be complicated by cavitation, necrosis, empyema, and bronchopleural fistula. Cavities in the lung parenchyma are the results of caseation and necrosis and are seen in cases of TB, fungal infections, and anaerobic infections. Fluffy and nodular infiltration with early cavitation in the upper lobes or the superior segments of the lower lobes are classic for TB and should be considered in every situation with these presentations (Figure 7). Mycotic infections are usually characterized by cavitation, necrosis, and pleural involvement. Hilar and mediastinal adenopathy, soft tissue involvement, and local and distal bony involvements are also features of mycotic infections.

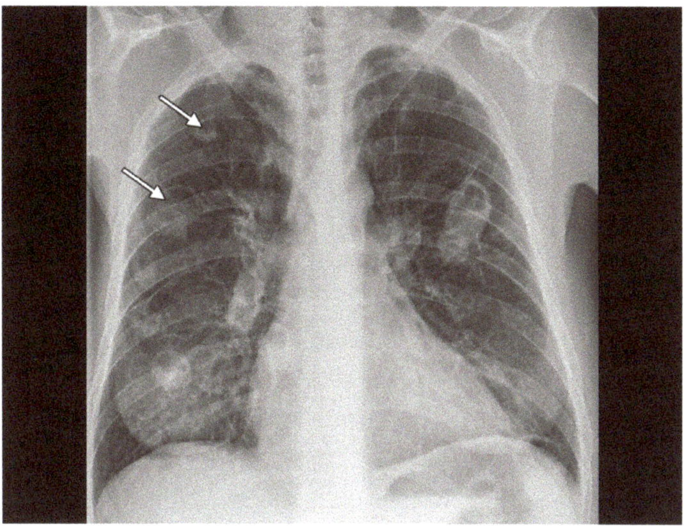

Figure 6: Bilateral multiple cavitary lesions, classic for septic pulmonary embolism and pneumonia due to hematogenous spread often caused by methicillin-resistant *Staphylococcus aureus* infection.

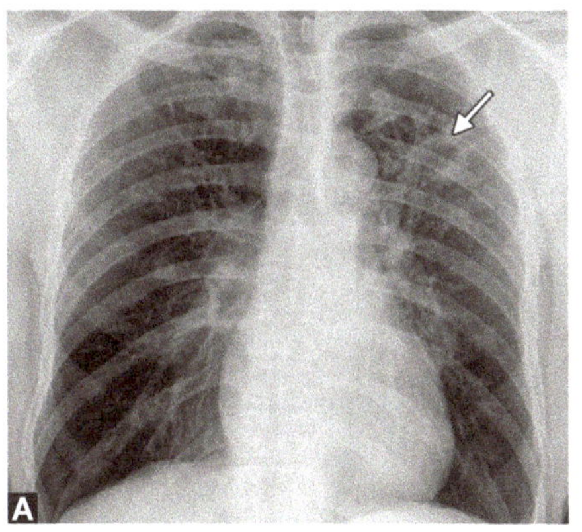

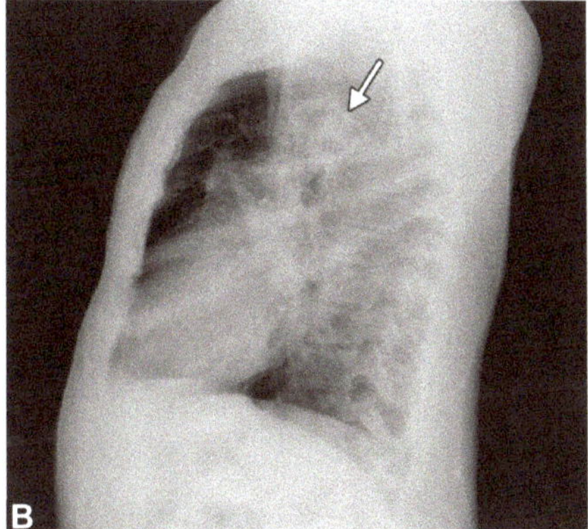

Figure 7: A, Posteroanterior and **B,** Lateral view of the chest X-ray showing bilateral apical nodular abnormalities with cavities in the left upper lobe highly suggestive of tuberculosis.

Clinicoradiographic Integration with Chest X-ray

Utility of Chest X-ray during the Initial Phase of Pneumonia

A normal chest radiograph is equally helpful especially in triaging febrile patients to look for another cause of patient's symptom complex. Noninfectious conditions like thromboembolic diseases should be considered especially if shortness of breath is associated with chest pain and hypoxia. In elderly patients, radiographic findings may be lagging the clinical findings often due to poor fluid status and the follow-up radiograph after adequate hydration becomes valuable. In elderly patients, underlying disorders like emphysema, pulmonary fibrosis, and cardiac failure play a role in diminishing diagnostic accuracy of chest radiographs. A population-based cohort study showed patients without radiographic findings had similar rates of identification of microorganisms in the blood, sputum, and a comparable mortality rate in suspected cases of pneumonia even in the absence of radiographic findings of pneumonia.[13]

Clinical radiographic integration is a key ingredient in the etiological diagnosis of pneumonia. Incidence of certain infections varies wildly because of geographic predilection and seasonal predisposition to certain microbial infections. Travel history, occupation, associated medical condition, and the medication history helps the clinician and the radiologists to come up with the cause of infectious or inflammatory disorder in a specific patient. It is important to know the patients' geographic location in the antibiotic management for healthcare associated pneumonia.[14,15] Experienced clinicians and the radiologists can predict suspected organisms with the incorporation of clinical history as outlined in table 1.[16]

Utility of Chest X-ray during the Treatment Phase of Pneumonia

Following treatment, radiographic improvement is noted within 10 days. Ninety percent of patients show radiographic resolution within 4 weeks. Resolution is slow in patients over the age of 50 years.[17,18] On follow-up, chest radiographs if the abnormality persists or if there are evidence of complications advanced imaging with CT scans or further interventions are warranted in the assessment of pneumonia.[19] Delayed resolution or progression of parenchymal abnormality can be due to ineffective treatment.[17,20]

Table 1: Classic Radiographic Findings and Causative Organisms

Radiographic findings	Causative organisms
Lobar consolidation	*Streptococcus pneumoniae, Legionella* spp.
Lobar enlargement (Bulging Fissure sign)	*Klebsiella Pneumoniae*
Atypical pneumonia	Mycoplasma, Chlamydia, *Legionella* spp.
Bronchopneumonia	*Hemophillus influenza, Branhamella, Staphylococcus*, Gram-negative organisms
Cavitation	Staphylococci, group B streptococci, anaerobic infections, tuberculosis, mycotic infections
Interstitial pneumonia	*Mycoplasma*, viral infections, *Pneumocystis jirovecii*

COMPUTED TOMOGRAPHY SCAN FINDINGS IN INFECTIOUS PNEUMONIA

Computed tomography scanning is very sensitive and superior imaging modality to chest radiograph because it shows precise anatomy of the alveolar-interstitial units and the small airways where the changes due to infection and inflammation occur.[8,21] Computed tomography scanning in detecting early pulmonary parenchymal abnormalities with well-known specific CT scan patterns early in the course of infection is very helpful in distinguishing various forms of pneumonias. In a retrospective analysis of over 2,000 patients with suspected respiratory infections in an emergency center, 27% patients had CT scan detected abnormalities when the chest radiographs were normal.[22] In a setting where the clinical evidence points to respiratory infection and the radiograph is negative, empiric antibiotic treatment with further imaging studies are acceptable.[22] Several CT findings are seen (Table 2) in lower respiratory tract infections which are due to the imaging abnormality caused by early pathological changes of inflammation, edema, cellular infiltrates and the changes due to tissue destruction.

Computed Tomography Scan Patterns and Signs in Uncomplicated Pneumonia

Alveolar Pattern: Parenchymal Attenuation, Ground-glass Opacification and Dense Consolidation with Air Bronchogram

Ground-glass opacification (GGO) is a distinct and early abnormal CT scan finding, appearing like a fine curtain over the alveoli and respiratory bronchioles before the blood vessels are obliterated by the density (Figure 8). Air-filled alveolar ducts and small airways can be seen. Ground-glass opacification is synonymous with air-alveologram and air-acinogram which will lead to denser consolidation eventually. Ground-glass opacification is a subnodular opacity and this density which does not obliterate the vascular shadows is due to consolidation of the alveoli and respiratory bronchioles. Ground-glass opacification pattern is usually suggestive of an alveolar filling process which can be due to infectious or noninfectious causes.[23] Early involvement of bronchiolar epithelium and

Table 2: Computed Tomography Findings in Pneumonia
Parenchymal attenuation, ground glass opacity, and consolidation
Nodules and tree in bud opacities
Inter lobar septal thickening
Bronchiolar and bronchial wall thickening

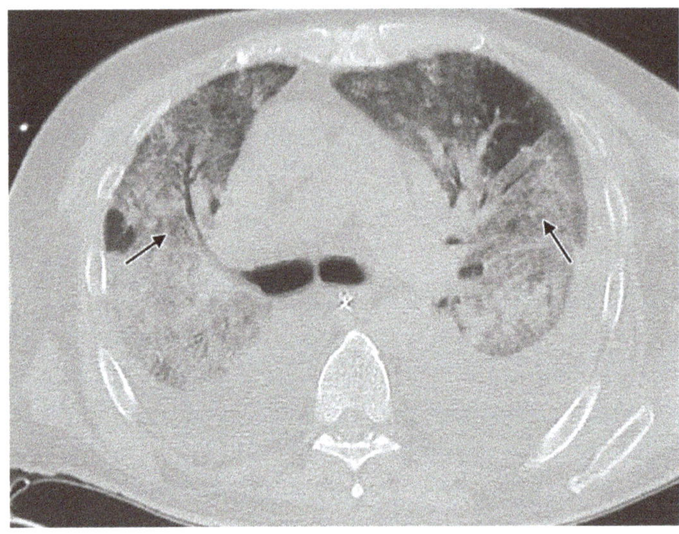

Figure 8: Computed tomography scan is showing bilateral ground-glass opacities with classic air bronchogram (black arrows), additionally there is bilateral pleural effusion.

Table 3: Common Causes of Ground-glass Opacity Pattern
• Infectious process, i.e., pneumocystis
• Acute alveolar process: Edema, hemorrhage, and diffuse alveolar damage
• Chronic interstitial process: Interstitial pneumonias, cryptogenic organizing pneumonia
• Resolving consolidation with restoration of airflow
• Other causes: Drug induced lung diseases, hypersensitivity pneumonitis, malignancy

peribronchial tissue with mononuclear infiltration of the alveolar septa leads to GGO and is indicative of interstitial pattern due to infection by PJP, mycoplasma, or viruses.[24] Ground-glass opacification is very nonspecific and can be seen in many infectious and noninfectious conditions[8] (Table 3).

Airspace consolidation is denser with obliteration of vasculature and can be segmental, lobar, or multilobar. A confluent density with air bronchogram is diagnostic for a classic bacterial pneumonia often caused by *S. Pneumoniae*, although can be seen with other infections as well. Though commonly seen with infection, adenocarcinoma, lymphoma, aspiration, cryptogenic organizing pneumonia, and nonobstructive atelectasis should be considered in the differential diagnosis of consolidation[25] (Figure 9).

Interstitial Pattern—Septal Thickening

Alveolar walls and the interlobular septa are thickened with edema leading to an interstitial pattern. This sensitive finding occurs from many causes of interstitial

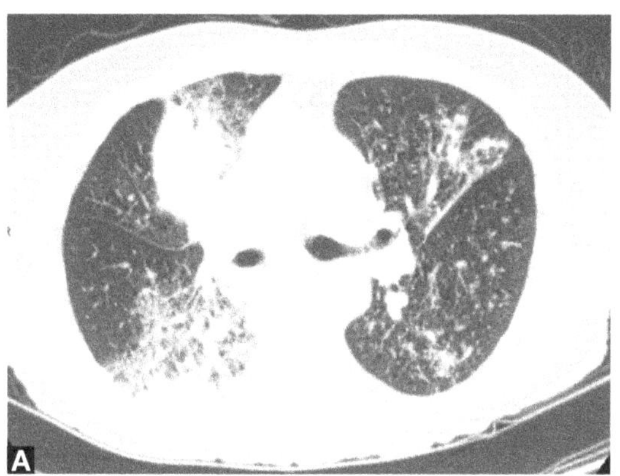

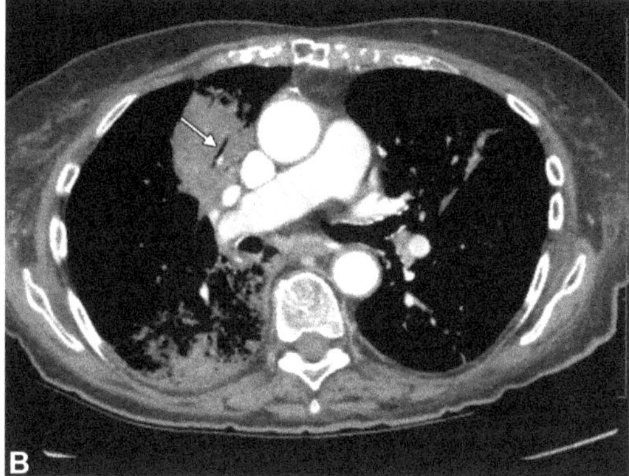

Figure 9: A, Lung window; **B,** mediastinal window of computed tomography showing dense mass like consolidation in UL, additionally LL is also showing consolidation with air-bronchograms (small white arrow).

edema and pathology. In early cases of mycoplasma pneumonia and many viral infections the bronchiolitis and interstitial involvement lead to bronchial wall and septal thickening. A strong clinical history and correlation is helpful in differentiating from a variety of noninfectious inflammatory disorder.

A characteristic pattern of GGO with septal thickening described originally in pulmonary alveolar proteinosis as crazy-paving sign is much more commonly seen in early cases of PJP (Figure 10). Crazy-paving pattern is also seen in pulmonary edema, pulmonary hemorrhage, pulmonary adenocarcinoma, lipoid pneumonia, and hypersensitivity pneumonitis.[25] In PJP, this pattern is due to alveolar exudative inflammation and the thickening of the interlobular septa due to edema.

Nodules and Tree and Bud Pattern

In a CT scan, a reticulonodular pattern is the predominant pattern in infectious and inflammatory disorders of the lung.[26] This pattern is formed by bronchial wall thickening leading to the bronchocentric nodules formed by the infectious and inflammatory exudate. The pleural surfaces are spared early in the infection. Tree-in-bud pattern is characteristic of infection with the centrilobular nodule and the thickening of the leading bronchiole with inspissated secretions (Figure 11).

Bronchopneumonia

A multifocal abnormality which begins as centrilobular nodules, exudative bronchiolitis, and bronchitis begin in the central airways. Though centrilobular nodular pattern can be the starting abnormality, alveolar and airway filling soon predominates in infectious pneumonia causing the bronchopneumonia pattern (Figure 12). A rapid spread of the infection with bronchial predominant

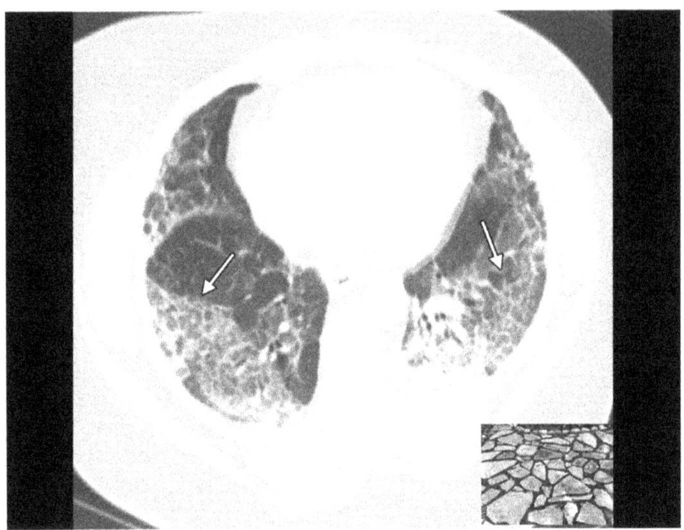

Figure 10: Computed tomography scan of lung bases showing acute and chronic interstitial changes and "crazy paving" pattern in a patient with possible *Pneumocystis jirovecii* pneumonia (Inserted image on right lower corner shows irregular pavement for comparison).

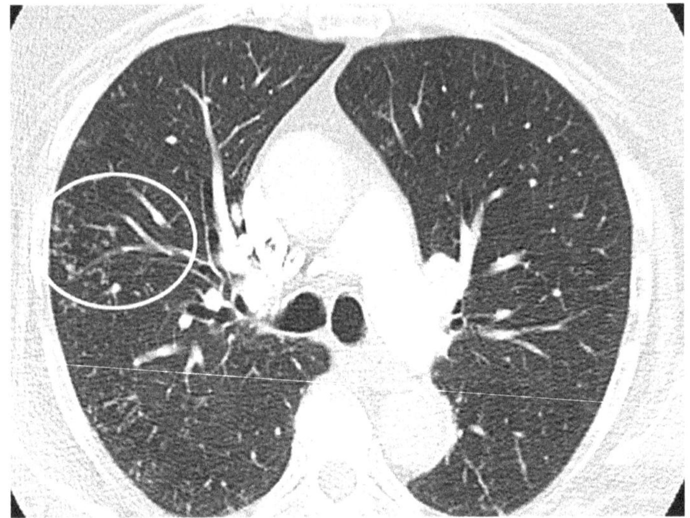

Figure 11: Tree-in-bud pattern in the peripheral lung fields usually suggestive of bronchiolitis caused by viral infection and *Mycobacterium* infection (like *Mycobacterium avium* complex).

consolidation without respecting the tissue plains and the lobes with early involvement of pleura is a feature of infection by staphylococci, *Pseudomonas aeruginosa*, and other gram-negative organisms. Nosocomial pneumonia, aspiration

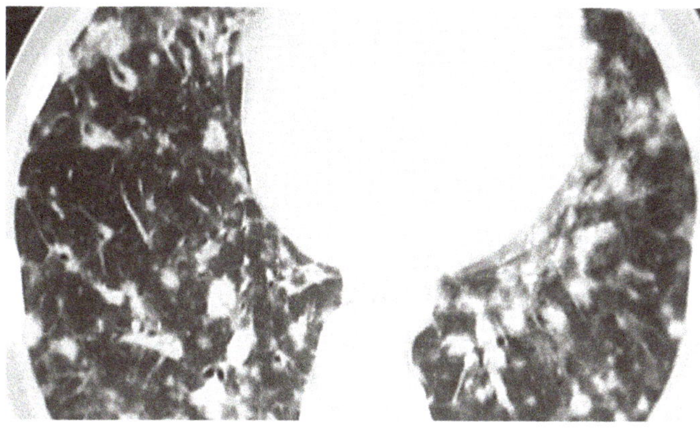

Figure 12: Computed tomography scan showing bronchopneumonia; multiple, bilateral, multilobar opacities; some of them are also showing early cavity formation, classic for septic pulmonary embolism mostly caused by methicillin-resistant *Staphylococcus aureus* infection.

pneumonia, and infections in immunocompromised patients also present with a bronchopneumonia pattern. Multifocal nodules, pneumatoceles, early cavitation, necrosis, and pleural effusion can be diagnostic of MRSA pneumonia.

Computed Tomography Scan Patterns and Signs in Complicated Pneumonia

Pneumonia can be complicated by cavitation, necrosis, empyema, and bronchopleural fistula. Pleuropulmonary complications like lung abscesses, empyema, and bronchopleural fistulas are detected early and often with the CT scan[26] (Figure 13). Classic CT scan findings of necrosis and cavities seen in aggressive gram-positive, gram-negative aerobic, anaerobic infections, mycotic, and mycobacterial infections are quite different from the common community-acquired pneumonia. Computed tomography scanning is a valuable imaging method in complex respiratory infections in detecting early necrosis, cavities (Figure 14), empyema, and bronchopleural fistula as a complication of pneumonia.

Abscesses are fluid filled cavities with a thick wall and the CT findings of air fluid levels along with the location of these lesions and the ability to discriminate the cavitary structures are extremely useful to confirm the diagnosis in the setting of infection and nonresolving pneumonia. Contrast CT scan is extremely helpful and the pleural enhancement with contrast is helpful in the management of pleuropulmonary complications like empyema which can occur during the course of pneumonia.[27,28] A "split pleural sign" is present when the thickened visceral and parietal pleura are identified in the presence of pleural effusion. Though,

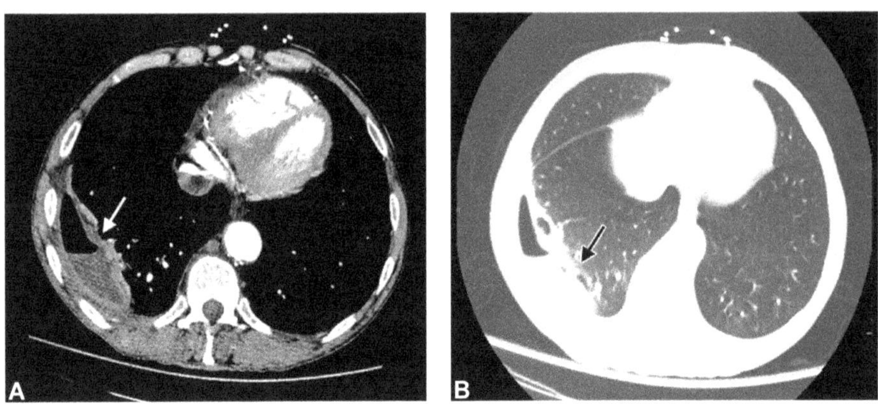

Figure 13: A, Computed tomography mediastinal windows show loculated hydropneumothorax (white arrow); **B,** Computed tomography lung window shows communicating bronchus (black arrow) with hydropneumothorax suggestive of bronchopleural fistula.

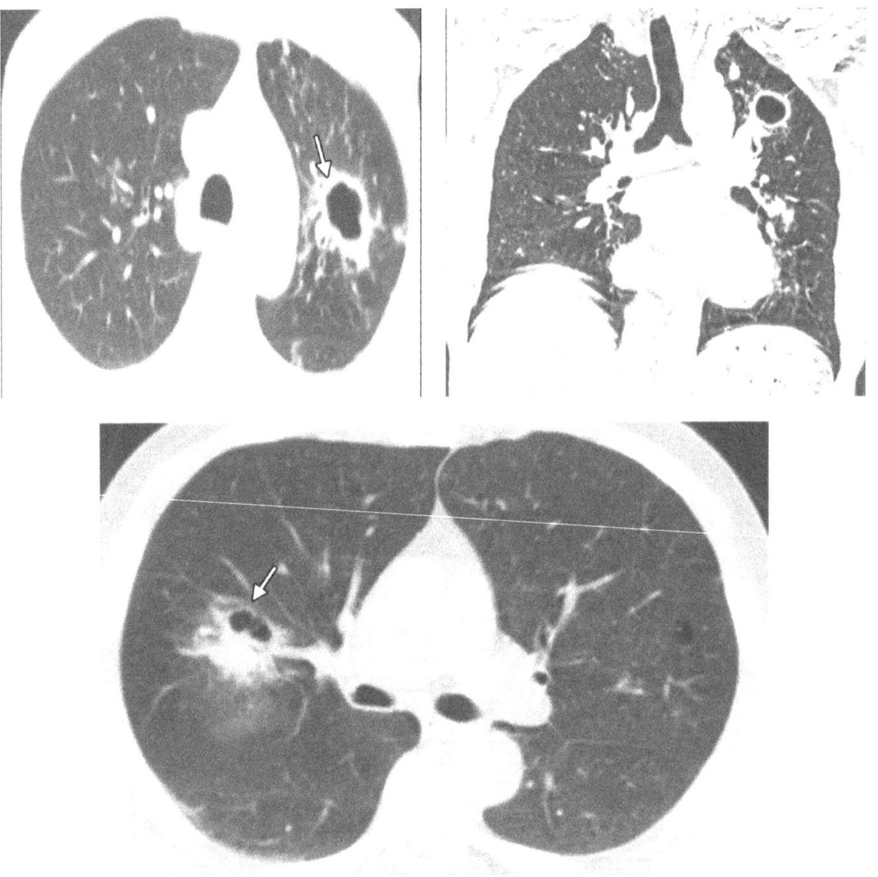

Figure 14: Computed tomography images showing right upper lobe and left lower lobe cavitary lesions with surrounding consolidations.

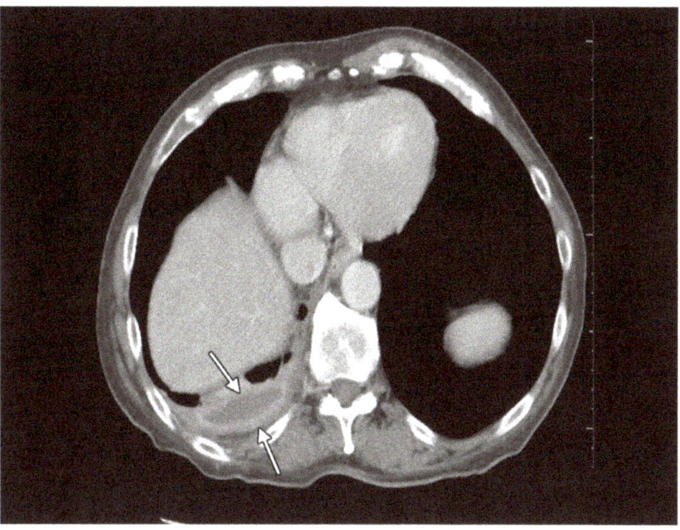

Figure 15: Pleural thickening, loculated effusion, and the "split pleural sign" of empyema.

nonspecific, a split pleural sign (Figure 15) was noted in 68% of cases in a series of 58 patients with empyema.[25,29,30] "Split pleural sign" is diagnostic of empyema in a setting of nonresolving pneumonia with persistent fever, chest pain, and cough.[25,29,30] Computed tomography scans are used to identify specific etiology in an expedited fashion which helps in targeted intervention with additional diagnostic procedures especially in immunocompromised patients.[27,28]

Other Computed Tomography Scan Findings

Random Nodules

Randomly distributed nodules represent hematogenous spread of infection, malignancy, or a noninfectious inflammatory disorder. This classic pattern is seen in miliary TB, mycotic infections, varicella pneumonia, and hematogenous metastasis.

Miliary Pattern

Miliary pattern is characterized by predominant centrilobular micronodules with branching septal pattern seen in CT scans (Figure 16). Though miliary TB jumps out as an all-important diagnostic consideration for miliary micronodular pattern, many other infectious and noninfectious conditions share this characteristic radiographic pattern listed in table 4.

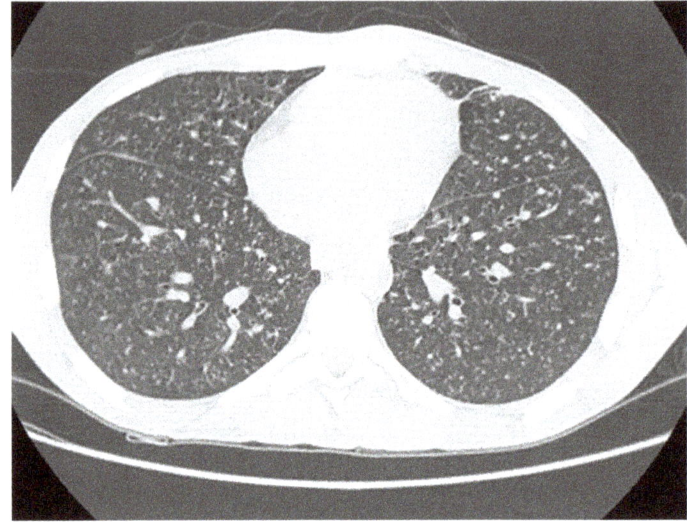

Figure 16: Computed tomography scan showing multiple (innumerable) small (millets like) nodules suggestive of miliary pattern.

Table 4: Causes of Miliary Nodules in Computed Tomography Scans

- Miliary tuberculosis
- Mycotic: Histoplasmosis, coccidioidomycosis, blastomycosis
- Sarcoidosis
- Miliary metastasis
- Viruses: Cytomegalovirus, herpes, varicella
- Kaposi's sarcoma
- Wegener's granulomatosis
- Lymphoma

Lymphadenopathy and Mass Lesions

Detection of associated findings of mass lesions, lymphadenopathy, and soft tissue involvement have become invaluable for clinicians in helping to identify complex infections like TB, mycotic infections and associated neoplastic processes.[31]

Halo Sign

Commuted tomographic finding of GGO adjacent to a denser nodule or a mass is known as "Halo sign" (Figure 17). This appearance is caused by a localized hemorrhage and should signal the diagnosis of invasive aspergillosis in an immunocompromised patient with neutropenia.[25,32,33] Halo sign was present in 90% of immunocompromised patients with pneumonia and neutropenia and

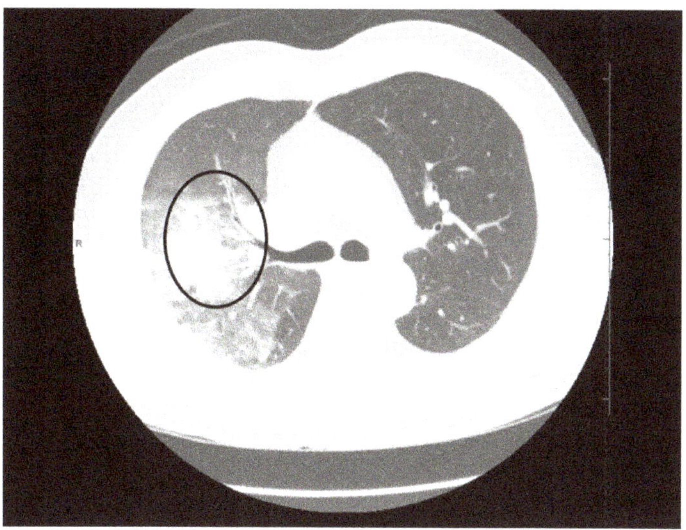

Figure 17: Computed tomography scan is showing dense consolidation with air-bronchogram (circle) surrounded by ground-glass opacity, known as "halo sign."

again emphasizes the importance of high-resolution computed tomography in this subset of patients.[34] Other causes of localized intraparenchymal hemorrhage like mucormycosis, candida, pseudomonas, herpes simplex, CMV infection, Wegener's granulomatosis, hemorrhagic metastasis, and Kaposi's sarcoma should be considered if Halo sign is present.[25]

Atelectasis

Classic segmental or lobar atelectasis is a rare finding of respiratory infections. Atelectasis indicates airway obstruction due to mucous plugging. Nonobstructive atelectasis has been described early in the course of respiratory infection and this could be due to poor pulmonary compliance of the involved segment or a lobe.

Clinicoradiographic Integration with Computed Tomography Scan

Computed tomography scanning has become a valuable imaging modality in detecting the etiology of infection in immunocompetent as well as immunocompromised hosts especially in human immunodeficiency virus/acquired immunodeficiency syndrome (HIV/AIDS) patients in whom infections can be complex and advanced at the time of presentation. Use of CT scanning has become a frontline approach in the evaluation of HIV/AIDS patients. With the classic and characteristic radiographic presentations in cases of infections notably by *Pneumocystis jirovecii, Mycobacterium tuberculosis*, nontuberculous mycobacteria, *Aspergillus*, and other invasive fungal organisms the role of CT imaging has become invaluable.[24] Computed tomography scanning is more sensitive and specific in predicting etiological agents in infections than plain radiographs.[24] Computed tomography scan findings and their diagnostic significances are given in table 5.

ULTRASONOGRAPHY IN THE DIAGNOSIS OF INFECTIOUS PNEUMONIA

For years air containing lung was considered as interference and created annoying artifacts during thoracic ultrasonography. With expertise in intensive care unit (ICU) and point of care examinations in the emergency centers ultrasonography has become an excellent additional imaging modality in the diagnosis of simple and complex pneumonias.[35,36] Systematic review and meta-analysis of ultrasound compared to CT scan and chest radiograph has shown a diagnostic accuracy of 88–95%.[37,38] Varying degrees of success has been reported in detecting consolidation with ultrasonography in adult patients with respiratory infections and studies show the sensitivity of the test around 90% and is comparable with chest radiography.[39]

Table 5: Computed Tomography Findings and Their Diagnostic Significance in Infectious and Inflammatory Disorders

Findings	Diagnostic significance
Ground glass opacification (GGO)	Early consolidation
Septal thickening	Edema of lobular and lobar septa
Tree in bud appearance	Bronchial wall thickening with centrilobular nodules
Halo sign	Perinodular hemorrhage or consolidation
Cavities	Tissue necrosis and abscess formation
Cysts	Thin walled cavities or pneumatoceles
Nodules	Denser areas of consolidation
Lymphadenopathy	Secondary to infection or inflammation
Air bronchogram	Consolidation with air filled airways
Pleural effusion	Involvement of pleural space
Diffuse pattern	Bronchopneumonia, acute respiratory distress syndrome
Atelectasis	Obstructed airways filled with exudates or mucoid impaction
Predominantly basilar involvement	Aspiration pneumonia

With the findings of fluid filled alveologram and the presence of broncho-aerogram in the right clinical setting, the diagnosis of pneumonic consolidation is confirmed in over 90% of cases.[40,41]

Consolidation is clearly identified as hypoechoic areas of varying size extending to the pleura associated with hyperechoic air bronchograms (Figure 18). Images of air-inlets are bronchograms similar to air-bronchograms in plain chest radiographs and air acinograms of CT scans. In addition, ultrasound images show fluid alveolograms and fluid bronchograms indicating the presence of exudates in alveoli and bronchioles. Color Doppler studies can be used to differentiate fluid filled airways from the blood vessels. Pleural effusions are noted in the dependent lung zones in up to 65% of pneumonia cases and are a sensitive and helpful finding in diagnosing pneumonia. Detection of the air bronchogram helps to differentiate between consolidation and atelectasis.[42,43] Ultrasonography helps to identify septations, loculations, and adhesions, which are features of complex pleural involvement due to empyema. Detection of the sliding lung phenomenon after thoracentesis is extremely helpful to rule out procedure related pneumothorax with great confidence.[37] Ultrasound procedure is repeatable and provides additional information, which is valuable in management of pneumonia in the emergency center and in the critical care units.[42] On the basis of studies showing a sensitivity of 85–95% and a specificity of 92%, many authors have proposed ultrasonography as the initial diagnostic procedure in the evaluation of pneumonia.[39,44-46] With emphasis of the use of thoracic ultrasound as a point of care examination and with improvement of the skills of dynamic ultrasonography by physician it is expected ultrasonography will be the initial imaging modality in the evaluation of pneumonia.

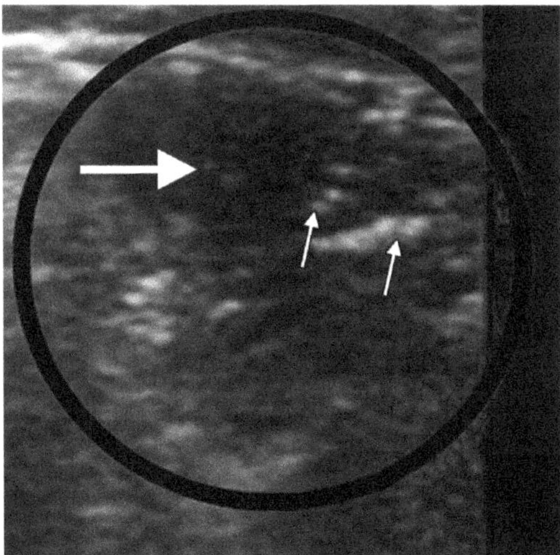

Figure 18: Lung ultrasound showing focal black hypoechoic area (large white arrow) surrounded by air-bronchogram (small white arrows) suggestive of pneumonia (black circle).

CONCLUSION

Ever since the original description of the use of chest radiography in the diagnosis of classic lobar pneumonia and cavitary TB, imaging has remained as the corner stone as a diagnostic procedure in detecting the etiology and in the subsequent clinical follow up for respiratory infections. With emerging infections by complex organisms and rapidly evolving sporadic and epidemic infections, radiological advances have met the challenge in helping the clinicians in the management of pneumonia. Advances in diagnostic and interventional radiology help the clinicians to manage patients with pneumonia with treatment options and the utilization of critical care resources.

Editor's Comment

Pneumonia is diagnosed on the basis of clinical symptoms and a radiological opacity. Hence, chest radiograph is considered as a gold standard investigation in pneumonia. Now due to the advancement in imaging techniques, computed tomography thorax and ultrasound also help the clinician to identify and manage pneumonia and its complications effectively. Prompt radiographic evaluation of patients with pneumonia is of paramount importance to reduce the morbidity and mortality associated with the delay in the diagnosis and management of such cases. Plain chest radiograph is all the more important considering the fact that this is the most frequently prescribed investigation in the outpatient department all over the world. Most of the pneumonia cases can be identified through a plain radiograph of the chest. In addition to helping with the early diagnosis of pneumonia, chest radiograph helps to stratify the severity of pneumonia. Careful radiological evaluation also helps in the etiological diagnosis of pneumonia. Experienced clinicians and the radiologists can predict suspected organisms with the incorporation of clinical history. Computed tomography scanning is very sensitive and shows precise anatomy of the alveolar-interstitial units and the small airways where the changes due to inflammation occur. Computed tomography thorax and ultrasound are employed mostly when the pneumonia remains unresolved or when there are complications such as pleural effusion and cavitation. Advances in imaging and interventional procedures help to detect associated findings of mass lesions, lymphadenopathy, and soft tissue involvement. In this article, the authors present a comprehensive review of the role of the diagnostic imaging methods in the evaluation of patients with infectious pneumonia and associated complications.

Ravindran Chetambath

REFERENCES

1. Fleischner FG. The visible bronchial tree; a roentgen sign in pneumonic and other pulmonary consolidations. *Radiology.* 1948;50(2):184-9.
2. Fleischner F. Der sichtbare Bronchialbaum, ein differentialdiagnostisches Symptom im Röntgenbild der Pneumonie. *Fortschr Geb Roentgenstr.* 1927;36:319-23.
3. Mandell LA, Wunderink RG, Anzueto A, et al. Infectious Diseases Society of America/American Thoracic Society consensus guidelines on the management of community-acquired pneumonia in adults. *Clin infect Dis.* 2007;44 Suppl 2:S27-72.
4. McLoud TC. Thoracic radiology: The requisites. St. Louis: Mosby; 1998.
5. Boersma WG, Daniels JM, Lowenberg A, et al. Reliability of radiographic findings and the relation to etiologic agents in community-acquired pneumonia. *Respir Med.* 2006;100(5):926-32.
6. Hopstaken RM, Witbraad T, van Engelshoven JM, et al. Inter-observer variation in the interpretation of chest radiographs for pneumonia in community-acquired lower respiratory tract infections. *Clin Radiol.* 2004;59(8):743-52.
7. Woodhead M, Blasi F, Ewig S, et al. Guidelines for the management of adult lower respiratory tract infections. *Eur Respir J.* 2005;26(6):1138-80.
8. Reynolds JH, Banerjee AK. Imaging pneumonia in immunocompetent and immunocompromised individuals. *Curr Opin Pulm Med.* 2012;18(3):194-201.
9. Tarver RD, Teague SD, Heitkamp DE, et al. Radiology of community-acquired pneumonia. *Radiol Clin North Am.* 2005;43(3):497-512.
10. Henzler T, Meyer M, Kalenka A, et al. Image findings of patients with H1N1 virus pneumonia and acute respiratory failure. *Acad Radiol.* 2010;17(6):681-5.
11. Agarwal PP, Cinti S, Kazerooni EA. Chest radiographic and CT findings in novel swine-origin influenza A (H1N1) virus (S-OIV) infection. *AJR Am J Roentgenol.* 2009;193(6):1488-93.
12. Johkoh T. Imaging of idiopathic interstitial pneumonias. *Clin Chest Med.* 2008;29(1):133-47.
13. Basi SK, Marrie TJ, Huang JQ, et al. Patients admitted to hospital with suspected pneumonia and normal chest radiographs: Epidemiology, microbiology, and outcomes. *Am J Med.* 2004;117(5):305-11.
14. Hoffken G, Niederman MS. Nosocomial pneumonia: the importance of a de-escalating strategy for antibiotic treatment of pneumonia in the ICU. *Chest.* 2002;122(6):2183-96.
15. American Thoracic Society; Infectious Diseases Society of America. Guidelines for the management of adults with hospital-acquired, ventilator-associated, and healthcare-associated pneumonia. *Am J Respir Crit Care Med.* 2005;171(4):388-416.
16. Meholic A, Ketai L, Lofgren R. Fundamentals of chest radiology. Philadelphia; Saunders: 1996.
17. Sharma S, Maycher B, Eschun G. Radiological imaging in pneumonia: Recent innovations. *Curr Opin Pulm Med.* 2007;13(3):159-69.
18. Johnson JL. Slowly resolving and nonresolving pneumonia. Questions to ask when response is delayed. *Postgrad Med.* 2000;108(6):115-22.
19. Bruns AH, Oosterheert JJ, El Moussaoui R, et al. Pneumonia recovery: discrepancies in perspectives of the radiologist, physician and patient. *J Gen Intern Med.* 2010;25(3):203-6.
20. Dean NC, Bateman KA, Donnelly SM, et al. Improved clinical outcomes with utilization of a community-acquired pneumonia guideline. *Chest.* 2006;130(3):794-9.
21. Syrjala H, Broas M, Suramo I, et al. High-resolution computed tomography for the diagnosis of community-acquired pneumonia. *Clin Infect Dis.* 1998;27(2):358-63.
22. Hayden GE, Wrenn KW. Chest radiograph vs. computed tomography scan in the evaluation for pneumonia. *J Emerg Med.* 2009;36(3):266-70.
23. Raoof S, Amchentsev A, Vlahos I, et al. Pictorial essay: Multinodular disease: A high-resolution CT scan diagnostic algorithm. *Chest.* 2006;129(3):805-15.
24. Beigelman-Aubry C, Godet C, Caumes E. Lung infections: The radiologist's perspective. *Diagn Interv Imaging.* 2012;93(6):431-40.

25. Walker CM, Abbott GF, Greene RE, et al. Imaging pulmonary infection: classic signs and patterns. *AJR Am J Roentgenol.* 2014;202(3):479-92.
26. Ketai L, Jordan K, Busby KH. Imaging infection. *Clin Chest Med.* 2015;36(2):197-217.
27. Kearney SE, Davies CW, Davies RJ, et al. Computed tomography and ultrasound in parapneumonic effusions and empyema. *Clin Radiol.* 2000;55(7):542-7.
28. Arenas-Jimenez J, Alonso-Charterina S, Sanchez-Paya J, et al. Evaluation of CT findings for diagnosis of pleural effusions. *Eur Radiol.* 2000;10(4):681-90.
29. Kuhlman JE, Singha NK. Complex disease of the pleural space: Radiographic and CT evaluation. *Radiographics.* 1997;17(1):63-79.
30. Stark DD, Federle MP, Goodman PC, et al. Differentiating lung abscess and empyema: Radiography and computed tomography. *AJR Am J Roentgenol.* 1983;141(1):163-7.
31. Aujesky D, Fine MJ. The pneumonia severity index: A decade after the initial derivation and validation. *Clin Infect Dis.* 2008;47 Suppl 3:S133-9.
32. Hansell DM, Bankier AA, MacMahon H, et al. Fleischner Society: Glossary of terms for thoracic imaging. *Radiology.* 2008;246(3):697-722.
33. Pinto PS. The CT Halo sign. *Radiology.* 2004;230(1):109-10.
34. Caillot D, Couaillier JF, Bernard A, et al. Increasing volume and changing characteristics of invasive pulmonary aspergillosis on sequential thoracic computed tomography scans in patients with neutropenia. *J Clin Oncol.* 2001;19(1):253-9.
35. Pelleciah C, Mayo PH. Ultrasound evaluation of the lung. Clinical chest ultrasound: From the ICU to the bronchoscopy suite. Progress in Respiratory Research. Basel: Karger; 2009.
36. Lichtenstein DA, Lascols N, Meziere G, Gepner A. Ultrasound diagnosis of alveolar consolidation in the critically ill. *Intensive Care Med.* 2004;30(2):276-81.
37. Alzahrani SA, Al-Salamah MA, Al-Madani WH, et al. Systematic review and meta-analysis for the use of ultrasound versus radiology in diagnosing of pneumonia. *Crit Ultrasound J.* 2017;9(1):6.
38. Long L, Zhao HT, Zhang ZY, et al. Lung ultrasound for the diagnosis of pneumonia in adults: A meta-analysis. *Medicine.* 2017;96(3):e5713.
39. Bourcier JE, Braga S, Garnier D. Lung ultrasound will soon replace chest radiography in the diagnosis of acute community-acquired pneumonia. *Curr Infect Dis Rep.* 2016;18(12):43.
40. Reissig A, Kroegel C. Sonographic diagnosis and follow-up of pneumonia: A prospective study. *Respiration.* 2007;74(5):537-47.
41. Reissig A, Kroegel C. Diagnosis of pulmonary embolism and pneumonia using trans thoracis sonography. Clinical chest ultrasound: From the ICU to the bronchoscopy suite. Progress in Respiratory Research. Basel: Karger; 2009.
42. Chavez MA, Shams N, Ellington LE, et al. Lung ultrasound for the diagnosis of pneumonia in adults: A systematic review and meta-analysis. *Respir Res.* 2014;15:50.
43. Benci A, Caremani M, Menchetti D, et al. Sonographic diagnosis of pneumonia and bronchopneumonia. *Eur J Ultrasound.* 1996;4(3):169-76.
44. Parlamento S, Copetti R, Di Bartolomeo S. Evaluation of lung ultrasound for the diagnosis of pneumonia in the ED. *Am J Emerg Med.* 2009;27(4):379-84.
45. Pagano A, Numis FG, Visone G, et al. Lung ultrasound for diagnosis of pneumonia in emergency department. *Intern Emerg Med.* 2015;10(7):851-4.
46. Volpicelli G, Mussa A, Garofalo G, et al. Bedside lung ultrasound in the assessment of alveolar-interstitial syndrome. *Am J Emerg Med.* 2006;24(6):689-96.

World Clin Pulm Crit Care Med. 2019;6(1):49-60.

Severity Assessment of Pneumonia

*Vivek Jayaschandran MD, Girish B Nair MD FACP FCCP

Department of Internal Medicine, Division of Pulmonary and Critical Care, William Beaumont Hospital
Oakland University School of Medicine, Royal Oak, Michigan, USA

ABSTRACT

Severe pneumonia is associated with high mortality and can occur in patients with both community-acquired pneumonia as well as with nosocomial pneumonia. Early recognition of severe illness can reduce mortality. Once recognized, severe pneumonia should be treated promptly, and delayed transfer to the intensive care unit (ICU) is associated with poor outcomes. Pneumonia risk stratification using prediction tools such as the Pneumonia Severity Index (PSI), CURB-65, SMART-COP, or American Thoracic Society (ATS) criteria can be used to help assess mortality risk and with decision on site of care. Biomarkers are being increasingly used as adjunctive tools along with severity scores to predict mortality risk and duration of antibiotics. This article summarizes the common risk predictor tools used in hospitalized community-acquired pneumonia patients.

INTRODUCTION

Pneumonia is a leading cause of septic shock and mortality worldwide.[1,2] Pneumonia related mortality increases to more than 10% in hospitalized patients, and can exceed 30% in those requiring intensive care unit (ICU) level of care.[3-5] Pneumococcal pneumonia related hospitalization is projected to increase 96% by 2040 in the United States alone, with an estimated increase of $2.5 billion annually in health care expenditure.[6] The elderly account for a disproportionate number of critically ill pneumonia patients, partly due to increased comorbid illness and a higher mortality compared to younger patients.

*Corresponding author
Email: vivek.jayaschandran@beaumont.edu

Severe pneumonia can occur in patients presenting from the community [community-acquired pneumonia (CAP)] or in patients developing pneumonia hospitalized for other reasons (nosocomial pneumonia). Patients who acquire severe pneumonia often have an excessive immune response to infection that is not localized to the initial site of lung infection or infection with multidrug resistant bacteria that is not responding to conventional antibiotics. Although, the majority of patients are cared for in the outpatient setting, the cost of care and overall mortality is higher among hospitalized patients compared to outpatients.

Accurate risk stratification and site of care decision are crucial initial steps in the assessment of patients with pneumonia. Any delay in appropriate antibiotic administration or ICU admission is associated with worse outcomes.[7,8] Unfortunately, clinical judgment alone has been shown to be a less useful predictor for assessing mortality risk in pneumonia patients evaluated in the emergency department (ER).[9] Current guidelines support the use of objective risk assessment tools to help determine the risk of mortality.[10,11] In this article, the authors discuss the significance of severity assessment in CAP and the various prognostic scoring systems currently available for clinical use.

RISKS STRATIFICATION IN SEVERE COMMUNITY-ACQUIRED PNEUMONIA

Several clinical and laboratory features predict poor outcomes in patients with CAP. In a study including 21,223 medicare patients, inhospital mortality was higher in patients requiring mechanical ventilation on admission, had bacteremia, hypotension (systolic blood pressure <90 mm Hg), respiratory rate of greater than 30/min, pH of less than 7.35, and renal failure.[3] Other risk factors for poor outcomes include advanced age (>65 years), pre-existing chronic illness, the absence of fever on admission, respiratory rate greater than 30 breaths/min, diastolic or systolic hypotension, elevated blood urea nitrogen [blood urea nitogen (BUN) >19.6 mg/dL], profound leukopenia or leukocytosis, inadequate antibiotic therapy, need for mechanical ventilation, hypoalbuminemia, and infection with "high-risk" organisms (type-III pneumococcus, *S. aureus*, gram-negative bacilli, aspiration organisms, or postobstructive pneumonia).[10] In a meta-analysis of 33,148 patients with CAP, the risk of mortality was increased in patients with pleuritic chest pain, hypothermia, hypotension, tachypnea, bacteremia, leukopenia, multilobar infiltrates on chest X-ray, and with male sex than females or if they have comorbid conditions, such as diabetes mellitus, neoplastic disease, or neurological dysfunction.[5]

Mortality associated with pneumonia is increased with a higher severity of illness on admission, need for ICU care, and the presence of multilobar infiltrates, but late mortality (after at least 3 days) was reduced if the blood cultures were negative, antibiotic therapy was consistent with guidelines, and if an etiologic agent was identified.[12] In a prospective study of 1,666 patients with severe pneumonia from 17 different countries, factors related with increased mortality at 28 days and at 6 months were high APACHE (Acute Physiology and Chronic Health Evaluation) II scores, low hematocrit and need for mechanical ventilation. Low pH on arterial blood gas analysis predicted early mortality.[4] In another study, investigators noted an increased mortality in patients who required mechanical ventilation after 4 or more days after the onset of CAP (28 vs. 51%, $p = 0.03$) than those who were identified to have respiratory failure, and mechanically ventilated within 72 hours of onset.[13] Delay in treatment or admission to the ICU can lead to higher rates of complications and increased mortality.[14,15]

Unfortunately, there is no uniform definition for severe pneumonia. It is clear from the above that severity of illness on admission, physiologic derangements, presence of comorbid conditions, and delay in initiation of appropriate antimicrobial therapy or mechanical ventilation affects mortality in hospitalized CAP patients (outpatient, hospital ward, or ICU). Several scoring systems were developed and validated over the last several years to help identify patients with severe pneumonia.

SEVERITY SCORES IN COMMUNITY-ACQUIRED PNEUMONIA

Recognizing the significance of pneumonia severity assessment, Infectious Disease Society of America and American Thoracic Society (IDSA/ATS) guidelines have incorporated risk stratification as a focal point in pneumonia management. Pneumonia Severity Index and British Thoracic Society's CURB-65 were the initial scoring systems developed to determine the risk of mortality and need for hospitalization.

Pneumonia Severity Index

The PSI utilizes a 20 point score to stratify patients into 5 categories based on 30 day mortality. The tool was developed in 1990s from a large data set of 14,199 CAP patients to identify those with low-risk of dying and safely be discharged home to receive outpatient treatment.[9] The risk assessment involves a two-step process. The first step uses variables immediately available to the physician such as age, co-existing conditions, and physical examination findings. This ensures that patients belonging to risk class 1 who have the lowest risk of 30 day mortality are identified early. Step 2 involves assigning points to variables including three demographic parameters, five comorbid conditions, five physical examination findings, and seven laboratory/imaging findings for patients who do not fall in the risk category 1. The cumulative score is then used to stratify patients into risk classes 2–5. Patients in classes IV (30-day mortality risk of 4–10%) and V (27% risk of death at 30 days) are usually admitted to the hospital and often to the ICU. Those in low-risk classes I and II are often treated as outpatients. In a meta-analysis comparing PSI, CURB-65, and CRB-65, all three tools performed well on 30 day mortality assessment, but PSI had the highest predictive accuracy (AUC 0.81).[16]

Despite being an excellent predictor of 30 day mortality, PSI score lacks ability to accurately predict ICU level care in CAP patients.[17] Pneumonia Severity Index score is influenced heavily by advanced age and presence of comorbid conditions and in contrast underestimate severity of illness in a young patient without comorbid conditions. An 81-year-old male with chronic kidney disease automatically falls in risk category 4, even if they do not have any other adverse prognostic factors; whereas a young patient with no comorbid conditions but significant physiological derangements will be categorized as a lower class. Further, it is cumbersome for physicians to go through an exhaustive list of variables to risk stratify patients, especially in the emergency room.

CURB-65

Recognizing the shortcomings of PSI, the British Thoracic Society proposed CURB-65 using five variables—confusion, urea >7 mmol/L, respiratory rate ≥30/min, systolic blood pressure (BP) less than 90 mm Hg or diastolic BP less than 60 mm Hg and age greater than 65 years.[18] One point is assigned for the presence of each of the component variable and cumulative score determines the overall CAP severity. A score of 0–1 suggests low-risk of dying and the patient can be managed as outpatient. Hospitalization is recommended for a score of 2 and strongly recommended for score of 3 or more (mortality risk of 40–57%). The simplicity of the score makes this tool very ideal for initial prognostication and multiple studies have demonstrated that it performs as well as PSI. CURB-65 is a simple tool, but as with PSI, CURB-65 has limitations with predicting the need for ICU stay. CURB-65 relies much on the initial vitals and does not measure physiological parameters of oxygenation or consider comorbid conditions.[19]

CRB-65 is a modification of CURB-65 that eliminates BUN level as a component variable and is mostly aimed at-risk stratifying CAP patients in an outpatient setting. CRB-65 is comparable to CURB-65 and PSI in predicting 30-day mortality. A meta-analysis of 40 studies demonstrated CURB-65 and CRB-65 to be superior to PSI in identifying high-risk patients, while PSI was superior in identifying low-risk patients.[16] An expanded version of CURB-65 that includes the three additional variables: platelet count less than 100 × 10(9)/L, lactate dehydrogenase levels more than 230 U/L, and albumin less than 3.5 g/dL was recently shown to have improved accuracy in identifying higher-mortality risk among hospitalized CAP patients.[20]

As mentioned above, both CURB-65 and CRB-65 scores do not account for hypoxemia, the major physiological impairment is related with pneumonia in the risk assessment. Three scores, namely, A-DROP, CORB, and DS-CRB 65 were designed to address this issue.

A-DROP

A-DROP was developed by the Japanese Respiratory Society in 2005, uses five variables to stratify CAP risk.[21] Essentially it is a modification of CURB-65 with inclusion of hypoxemia as a variable in place of respiratory rate and with different gender-based thresholds for age in risk assessment. The sensitivity, specificity, and 30 day mortality predictive value of the A-DROP scoring tool is similar to CURB-65.[22]

CORB

Buising et al., derived "CORB" as a simple predictive tool that does not require invasive testing, and removes bias regarding patient age.[23] The CORB tool does not use variables of age and BUN levels, but with the addition of oxygen saturation as a variable in the risk calculation. In both the derivation and validation cohort, risks of mortality and/or requirement for ventilatory or inotropic support were: systolic blood pressure less than 90 mm Hg [odds ratio (OR) 3.49]; acute confusion (OR 5.48); SaO_2 less than or equal to 90% (OR 3.49); and respiratory rate more than or equal to 30/min (OR 2.65).

DS-CRB 65

Dwyer et al. developed the "DS-CRB 65" criteria to improve the sensitivity and negative predictive value of CRB-65 by adding 1 point (D criterion) for the presence of any underlying disease according to the PSI rule, and 1 point if SaO_2 was less than 90% (S criterion).[24] A large multicenter validation of DS-CRB-65 showed that D criterion significantly improved mortality prediction whereas the S-criterion helped in better identification of patients needing invasive mechanical ventilation, vasopressor support or ICU care.[25]

INTENSIVE CARE UNIT LEVEL OF CARE

Any delay with ICU admission is related with increased mortality in severe CAP patients. Other than the DS-CRB-65, the severity scoring systems mentioned thus far does not accurately categorize patients at-risk of invasive mechanical ventilation or need for vasopressor requirements (MV/VS). The IDSA/ATS criteria for severe CAP, Risk of Early Admission to the ICU Index (REA-ICU), Australian SMART-COP scoring system, and the PIRO scoring system (predisposition, insult, response, and organ dysfunction) were developed to help define mortality risk in patients with severe pneumonia and need for ICU.

American Thoracic Society/Infectious Disease Society of America Criteria

American Thoracic Society criteria for defining severe CAP were originally published in 1993 and underwent further revisions in 2001 and 2007. The latest guidelines use a set of major and minor criteria to characterize severe CAP.[10] The presence of either of the two major criteria—invasive mechanical ventilation and hemodynamic compromise needing vasopressor support translated into a clinical diagnosis of severe CAP and ICU transfer for management. In the absence of the major criteria, presence of at least 3 of the 9 minor criteria predicted severe CAP and ICU admission is recommended. The minor criteria included respiratory rate more than 30 breaths/min, PaO_2/FiO_2 ratio less than 250, multilobar infiltrates, confusion/disorientation, uremia (BUN level >20 mg/dL), leukopenia (white blood cell count <4,000 cells/mm^3), thrombocytopenia (platelet count <100,000 cells/mm^3), hypothermia (core temperature <36°C), and hypotension requiring aggressive fluid resuscitation.[10]

The 2007 IDSA/ATS criteria have been extensively validated over the last several years. Valencia and associates noted in a study including 457 PSI class V patients; the modified ATS severity rule was more specific than the CURB-65 and had a high negative predictive value (91%) in predicting ICU admission.[17] The major criteria does not offer much clinical value in triaging as need for invasive mechanical ventilation or vasopressor use automatically qualifies for ICU transfer. Hence, a lot of emphasis has been given to the minor criteria and its ability to predict evolving severe CAP needing ICU admission. In a prospective study, including 1,062 patients with CAP, each of the 9 minor criteria was associated with increased risk of MV/VS and 30 day mortality.[26] The positive predictive value increased from 54 to 81% by using four rather than three minor criteria.[27] A meta-analysis testing the prognostic significance of each of the nine variables that constitute the minor criteria, simplified the score by excluding three variables—thrombocytopenia (<100,000 cells/mm^3), white blood cell count (<4,000 cells/mm^3), and hypothermia (<36°C)—that had less contribution to risk prognostication.[28] In that model, the simplified ATS minor criteria performed as well as the 2007 ATS minor criteria in terms of predicting mortality and ICU admission.

SMARTCOP

SMARTCOP is a simple, 8-variable tool that has been shown to accurately identify the need for ICU level care or more appropriately, the need for intensive respiratory or vasopressor support in CAP. Each variable is assigned a specific point: Low systolic blood pressure (1 point), multilobar chest radiography involvement (1 point), low albumin level (1 point), high respiratory rate (age adjusted; 1 point), tachycardia (1 point), confusion (1 point), poor oxygenation (age adjusted; 2 points), and low arterial pH (2 points).[29] Presence of more than 3 points identified 92% of patients who received intensive respiratory care or vasopressor support. In addition to patients admitted directly to the ICU, SMARTCOP was able to identify those patients who were initially admitted to the general ward, but later required ICU care. A simplified version of the tool called "SMRT-CO" eliminating the need for measuring PaO_2, albumin level, and arterial pH score is suitable for quick assessment of patients in primary care setting. This modified version assigns 2 points to major variables (low systolic blood pressure and hypoxia measured by pulse oximetry) and 1 point each for minor variables (confusion, tachycardia, tachypnea, and multilobar infiltrates). A SMRT-CO score of 2 points identified 82 (90.1%) of the 91 patients needing ICU care.

REA-ICU

Risk of Early Admission to the ICU Index (REA-ICU) was developed in order to identify patients at-risk of early (<3 days) deterioration and need for ICU care after initial hospitalization.[30] REA-ICU index uses 11 baseline characteristics to predict the need for ICU referral. Patients were risk stratified into four risk classes based on their cumulative score. The researchers excluded patients with obvious need for ICU admission, namely, patients requiring immediate circulatory or ventilator support and provide an objective assessment in the ER. REA-ICU index outperformed PSI, CURB-65, and severe community-acquired pneumonia (SCAP) scores in terms of predicting need for early ICU referral.[30,31]

SCAP Score

"SCAP score" or "Espana rule" used inhospital death, septic shock, and/or need for mechanical ventilation as endpoints to define severe CAP. Developed in 2006, in Spain, SCAP score relies on eight variables that are easily available at the time of ED admission to assess pneumonia severity.[32] A cumulative score of 10 was used as the cutoff to define severe CAP. In other words, presence of one major criterion or at least 2 minor criteria identified patients presenting with severe CAP. Essentially, SCAP score is an iteration of prediction scores such as PSI and

CURB-65 which recalculated the relative weight of the variables used in these previous scoring systems. SCAP uses a higher age cut off than CURB-65 and also includes the variables of pH, PaO_2/FiO_2 and extent of radiographic involvement. It is also a lighter version of PSI and using eight variables instead of twenty makes this tool more practical to use in the ED.

In the original derivation and validation cohorts, this tool could identify severe CAP with good accuracy (AUC of 0.92) and outperform modified ATS rule, CURB-65, and PSI.[32] A meta-analysis assessed the pooled performance of the SCAP score to predict ICU admission and found that sensitivity of the score was similar to what was noted in the original study (94%), but the specificity was lower (46 vs. 64%)[33] SCAP can also predict 30 day mortality in CAP with accuracy comparable to PSI and CURB-65. Additionally, SCAP score outperformed PSI and CURB-65 in identifying pneumonia patients at low-risk of mortality and less severe disease that could be managed outpatient.[34]

CAP-PIRO

CAP-PIRO uses the PIRO concept. The tool incorporates eight variables including comorbidities (chronic obstructive pulmonary disease, immuno-compromise), age more than 70 years, bacteremia, multilobar opacities in chest radiograph, shock, severe hypoxemia, acute renal failure, and acute respiratory distress syndrome obtained within 24 hours of ICU admission. Each variable was assigned one point and mortality risk was calculated based on the cumulative score. Patients were stratified in four levels of risk: (i) low, 0–2 points; (ii) mild, 3 points; (iii) high, 4 points; and (iv) very-high, 5–8 points.[35] Mild, high, and very-high risk levels were significantly associated with higher risk of death. CAP-PIRO can further stratify patients in PSI class V and differentiate patients requiring more intense care.

ROLE OF BIOMARKERS IN SEVERE COMMUNITY-ACQUIRED PNEUMONIA

Biomarkers are biologic characteristics that can be objectively measured and help distinguish normal from pathologic processes and measure response to therapy. In addition to prognostication, biomarkers were also proposed to be beneficial in CAP diagnosis, determining the need and duration of antibiotic therapy. Novel molecules studies included proinflammatory cytokines—tumor necrosis factor (TNF)-a, interleukin (IL)-1, IL-6, and acute-phase reactants-C-reactive protein (CRP), procalcitonin (PCT), and anti-inflammatory cytokines such as IL-1 receptor antagonist, IL-10 (Table 1).

Table 1: A List of the Best-studied Biomarkers for Pneumonia Severity Assessment

Biomarkers	Features
Acute phase reactants	
Procalcitonin	Produced by parenchymal cells like liver in response to bacterial toxins or proinflammatory cytokines but downregulated in viral infection[39]
C-reactive protein	Assists in recognition and elimination of pathogens by interacting with both humoral and cellular systems of inflammation
Hormones, prohormones	–
Copeptin	Copeptin is synthesized along with vasopressin from a precursor peptide and has been shown to predict severity of community-acquired pneumonia (CAP)
Pro-adrenomedullin	A vasodilator peptide hormone which plays a role in immunomodulation and bactericidal activity
Cortisol	Levels of the stress hormone, cortisol has been noted to be associated with severity of CAP and mortality
Atrial natriuretic peptide	A cardiac biomarker with prognostic significance in CAP

Most of the recent studies have focused on procalcitonin as a reliable hormokine that is specifically elevated in bacterial infections and more sensitive and specific than CRP in patients with pneumonia. A study that randomized 302 patients with radiographic CAP to receive either standard care or use serial PCT levels to guide antibiotic use showed that procalcitonin guidance reduced total antibiotic prescriptions on admission, and antibiotic treatment duration (median, 5 vs. 12 day; $p < 0.001$) compared to control group with no adverse outcomes in those not receiving therapy.[36] Furthermore, PCT can be used for risk stratification. Higher levels of PCT were noted in patients with increased mortality risk—PSI classes 4 and 5. Procalcitonin was also higher in patients with pneumonia complications and patients requiring ICU admission. Serial measurement of PCT can be useful in predicting the clinical course and an elevated PCT level on repeated measurement during hospital stay is associated with higher risk of mortality.[37] Combining biomarkers like CRP and PCT to risk prediction scores such as CURB-65 or PSI can improve mortality prediction in CAP.[38]

The use of PCT to determine antibiotic need does come with a few caveats. First it is not clear if PCT can distinguish between typical bacterial CAP and CAP due to atypical bacterial pathogens. Secondly, along with the nature of the pathogen, severity of illness can also influence PCT levels. During the

H1N1 epidemic, PCT levels certainly could distinguish most patients with pure viral infection from those with bacterial pneumonia, however, some patients with severe viral pneumonia had relatively high PCT levels that overlapped with levels found in patients with bacterial infection.[39] The ProRESP, ProCAP, and ProHOSP studies demonstrated that PCT, when combined with clinical judgment, can be used to determine the need for antibiotic therapy in CAP.[36,40]

CONCLUSION

Optimal site of care is a crucial initial step in the management of patients with pneumonia. Identification of high-risk patients requiring inpatient care and early stratification of inpatients as to those with severe pneumonia are pivotal steps in the management of severe pneumonia; thus, consideration will be given for aggressive management and ICU admission. It is imperative to combine the risk assessment with the subjective assessment of the patient before the final decision on site of care is made.

Editor's Comment

Risk stratification and site of care decision in community-acquired pneumonia is important in the management, influencing the patient outcomes and cost of treatment. Pneumonia severity index (PSI), the currently recommended tool, is cumbersome and time consuming as it is based on many variables. It is also considered that assessment based on PSI results in potential underestimation of severe pneumonia. CURB-65 and its simplified version CRB-65 are tools based on simple clinical approach not requiring sophisticated biochemical, immunological, or genetic data in the risk stratification of patients having acute potentially life-threatening condition. It can be applied easily in the outpatient clinic and predict 30 days mortality fairly accurately. There are many other tools which are validated for use. However, most of these tools assess community-acquired pneumonia only and often excluded special populations such as pneumonia in immunocompromised patients, aspiration pneumonia, etc. At the same, time physicians should be aware of the fact that any decisions about treatment settings must not rely exclusively on predictions of mortality alone. Other factors such as comorbidities, severe hypoxemia or hypercapnia, the extent of radiographic infiltrates, and pleural effusions are to be counted. The authors in this article lucidly describe almost all available risk stratification tools for both community-acquired pneumonia and ventilator-associated pneumonia, and substantiate these with adequate references.

Ravindran Chetambath

REFERENCES

1. Quenot JP, Binquet C, Kara F, et al. The epidemiology of septic shock in French intensive care units: The prospective multicenter cohort EPISS study. *Crit Care.* 2013;17:R65.
2. Phua J, Ngerng WJ, See KC, et al. Characteristics and outcomes of culture-negative versus culture-positive severe sepsis. *Crit Care.* 2013;17:R202.
3. Metersky ML, Waterer G, Nsa W, et al. Predictors of in-hospital vs postdischarge mortality in pneumonia. *Chest.* 2012;142:476-81.
4. Walden AP, Clarke GM, McKechnie S, et al. Patients with community acquired pneumonia admitted to European intensive care units: an epidemiological survey of the GenOSept cohort. *Crit Care.* 2014;18:R58.
5. Fine MJ, Smith MA, Carson CA, et al. Prognosis and outcomes of patients with community-acquired pneumonia. A meta-analysis. *JAMA.* 1996;275:134-41.
6. Wroe PC, Finkelstein JA, Ray GT, et al. Aging population and future burden of pneumococcal pneumonia in the United States. *J Infect Dis.* 2012;205:1589-92.
7. Kumar A, Roberts D, Wood KE, et al. Duration of hypotension before initiation of effective antimicrobial therapy is the critical determinant of survival in human septic shock. *Crit Care Med.* 2006;34:1589-96.
8. Iregui M, Ward S, Sherman G, et al. Clinical importance of delays in the initiation of appropriate antibiotic treatment for ventilator-associated pneumonia. *Chest.* 2002;122:262-8.
9. Fine MJ, Auble TE, Yealy DM, et al. A prediction rule to identify low-risk patients with community-acquired pneumonia. *N Engl J Med.* 1997;336:243-50.
10. Mandell LA, Wunderink RG, Anzueto A, et al. Infectious Diseases Society of America/American Thoracic Society consensus guidelines on the management of community-acquired pneumonia in adults. *Clin Infect Dis.* 2007;44 Suppl 2:S27-72.
11. Musher DM, Thorner AR. Community-acquired pneumonia. *N Engl J Med.* 2014;371:1619-28.
12. Garau J, Baquero F, Perez-Trallero E, et al. Factors impacting on length of stay and mortality of community-acquired pneumonia. *Clin Microbiol Infect.* 2008;14:322-9.
13. Hraiech S, Alingrin J, Dizier S, et al. Time to intubation is associated with outcome in patients with community-acquired pneumonia. *PloS One.* 2013;8:e74937.
14. Restrepo MI, Mortensen EM, Rello J, et al. Late admission to the ICU in patients with community-acquired pneumonia is associated with higher mortality. *Chest.* 2010;137:552-7.
15. Renaud B, Santin A, Coma E, et al. Association between timing of intensive care unit admission and outcomes for emergency department patients with community-acquired pneumonia. *Crit Care Med.* 2009; 37:2867-74.
16. Chalmers JD, Singanayagam A, Akram AR, et al. Severity assessment tools for predicting mortality in hospitalised patients with community-acquired pneumonia. Systematic review and meta-analysis. *Thorax.* 2010;65:878-83.
17. Valencia M, Badia JR, Cavalcanti M, et al. Pneumonia severity index class v patients with community-acquired pneumonia: characteristics, outcomes, and value of severity scores. *Chest.* 2007;132:515-22.
18. Lim WS, van der Eerden MM, Laing R, et al. Defining community acquired pneumonia severity on presentation to hospital: An international derivation and validation study. *Thorax.* 2003;58:377-82.
19. Nair GB, Niederman MS. Community-acquired pneumonia: An unfinished battle. *Med Clin North Am.* 2011;95:1143-61.
20. Liu JL, Xu F, Zhou H, et al. Expanded CURB-65: A new score system predicts severity of community-acquired pneumonia with superior efficiency. *Sci Rep.* 2016;6:22911.
21. Miyashita N, Matsushima T, Oka M, et al. The JRS guidelines for the management of community-acquired pneumonia in adults: An update and new recommendations. *Intern Med.* 2006;45:419-28.
22. Shindo Y, Sato S, Maruyama E, et al. Comparison of severity scoring systems A-DROP and CURB-65 for community-acquired pneumonia. *Respirology.* 2008;13:731-5.
23. Buising KL, Thursky KA, Black JF, et al. Identifying severe community-acquired pneumonia in the emergency department: a simple clinical prediction tool. *Emerg Med Australas.* 2007;19:418-26.

24. Dwyer R, Hedlund J, Darenberg J, et al. Improvement of CRB-65 as a prognostic scoring system in adult patients with bacteraemic pneumococcal pneumonia. *Scand J Infect Dis.* 2011;43:448-55.
25. Kolditz M, Ewig S, Schutte H, et al. Assessment of oxygenation and comorbidities improves outcome prediction in patients with community-acquired pneumonia with a low CRB-65 score. *J Intern Med.* 2015;278:193-202.
26. Chalmers JD, Taylor JK, Mandal P, et al. Validation of the Infectious Diseases Society of America/American Thoratic Society minor criteria for intensive care unit admission in community-acquired pneumonia patients without major criteria or contraindications to intensive care unit care. *Clin Infect Dis.* 2011;53:503-11.
27. Brown SM, Jones BE, Jephson AR, et al. Validation of the Infectious Disease Society of America/American Thoracic Society 2007 guidelines for severe community-acquired pneumonia. *Crit Care Med.* 2009;37: 3010-16.
28. Salih W, Schembri S, Chalmers JD. Simplification of the IDSA/ATS criteria for severe CAP using meta-analysis and observational data. *Eur Respir J.* 2014;43:842-51.
29. Charles PG, Wolfe R, Whitby M, et al. SMART-COP: A tool for predicting the need for intensive respiratory or vasopressor support in community-acquired pneumonia. *Clin Infect Dis.* 2008;47:375-84.
30. Renaud B, Labarere J, Coma E, et al. Risk stratification of early admission to the intensive care unit of patients with no major criteria of severe community-acquired pneumonia: Development of an international prediction rule. *Crit Care.* 2009;13:R54.
31. Labarere J, Schuetz P, Renaud B, et al. Validation of a clinical prediction model for early admission to the intensive care unit of patients with pneumonia. *Acad Emerg Med.* 2012;19:993-1003.
32. Espana PP, Capelastegui A, Gorordo I, et al. Development and validation of a clinical prediction rule for severe community-acquired pneumonia. *Am J Respir.* 2006;174:1249-56.
33. Marti C, Garin N, Grosgurin O, et al. Prediction of severe community-acquired pneumonia: A systematic review and meta-analysis. *Crit Care.* 2012;16:R141.
34. Espana PP, Capelastegui A, Quintana JM, et al. Validation and comparison of SCAP as a predictive score for identifying low-risk patients in community-acquired pneumonia. *J Infect.* 2010;60:106-13.
35. Rello J, Rodriguez A, Lisboa T, et al. PIRO score for community-acquired pneumonia: A new prediction rule for assessment of severity in intensive care unit patients with community-acquired pneumonia. *Crit Care Med.* 2009;37:456-62.
36. Christ-Crain M, Stolz D, Bingisser R, et al. Procalcitonin guidance of antibiotic therapy in community-acquired pneumonia: A randomized trial. *Am J Respir Crit Care Med.* 2006;174:84-93.
37. Lacoma A, Rodriguez N, Prat C, et al. Usefulness of consecutive biomarkers measurement in the management of community-acquired pneumonia. *Eur J Clin Microbiol Infect Dis.* 2012;31:825-33.
38. Huang DT, Weissfeld LA, Kellum JA, et al. Risk prediction with procalcitonin and clinical rules in community-acquired pneumonia. *Ann Emerg Med.* 2008;52:48-58.e2.
39. Upadhyay S, Niederman MS. Biomarkers: What is their benefit in the identification of infection, severity assessment, and management of community-acquired pneumonia? *Infect Dis Clin North Am.* 2013;27: 19-31.
40. Schuetz P, Christ-Crain M, Thomann R, et al. Effect of procalcitonin-based guidelines vs standard guidelines on antibiotic use in lower respiratory tract infections: The ProHOSP randomized controlled trial. *JAMA.* 2009;302:1059-66.

World Clin Pulm Crit Care Med. 2019;6(1):61-75.

Management of Pneumonia: An Overview

[1,*]Mohan Alladi MD DNB, [2]M Madhusudhan MD, [3]J Harikrishna MD

[1]Department of General Medicine, Sri Venkateswara Institute of Medical Sciences, Tirupati, Andhra Pradesh, India
[2]Department of Anesthesiology and Critical Care Medicine, Sri Venkateswara Institute of Medical Sciences, Tirupati, Andhra Pradesh, India
[3]Division of Pulmonary Critical Care Medicine, Sri Venkateswara Institute of Medical Sciences, Tirupati, Andhra Pradesh, India

ABSTRACT

Management of community-acquired pneumonia, hospital-acquired pneumonia, and ventilator-associated pneumonia aims at early diagnosis and institution of appropriate treatment. Deciding on which patients with pneumonia require intensive care unit admission is a key management decision especially in patients with severe comorbid conditions, malnutrition, and other risk factors for pneumonia. Disease severity scoring systems help in deciding on intensive care unit admission and assessing the prognosis. Initial empirical antibiotic treatment should cover both typical and atypical etiological causes. The antibiotic treatment should be modified to pathogen-specific treatment once bacterial culture and sensitivity testing results are available. Implementation of preventive strategies can help in reducing the risk of pneumonia.

INTRODUCTION

Pneumonia is an important public health problem, globally.[1-3] Clinical presentation of community-acquired pneumonia (CAP) varies in severity. Mild CAP (50–80%) can be managed with outpatient care. However, severe CAP (20–50%) may require hospital or intensive care unit (ICU) admission.[4] Hospital-acquired pneumonia (HAP) is the second most frequent nosocomial infection worldwide, affecting

*Corresponding author
Email: alladimohan@yahoo.com

0.5–1.7% of hospitalized patients.[5] In the ICU setting, ventilator-associated pneumonia (VAP) is the most common nosocomial infection and is the cause for 70–80% of HAP cases occurring in the ICU.[6]

Based on time of onset, HAP is divided in to early-onset, and late-onset HAP. Early-onset HAP occurs within the first 4 days of hospitalization. Common etiological pathogens causing early-onset HAP include "community" pathogens like *Streptococcus pneumoniae*, *Haemophilus influenzae*, and anaerobes. Late-onset HAP occurs after the fifth day of hospitalization. Organisms causing late-onset HAP include methicillin-resistant *Staphylococcus aureus* (MRSA), enteric gram-negative bacilli, *Pseudomonas aeruginosa*, nonfermenting aerobic gram-negative bacteria (e.g., *Acinetobacter baumannii* and Stenotrophomonas maltophilia); sometimes the etiology may be polymicrobial.[7] In comparison with early-onset HAP, late-onset HAP is associated with a mortality ranging from 30 to 70% and carries a poor prognosis. Factors associated with increased mortality in HAP in spite of adequate antimicrobial therapy and advances in supportive care include infection caused by multidrug-resistant (MDR) pathogens, delay in institution of specific, inappropriate/inadequate antibiotic therapy.[2,7,8]

MANAGEMENT

Management of pneumonia focuses on an early diagnosis and institution of appropriate therapy.

Diagnosis of Community-acquired Pneumonia

Clinical presentation of CAP may vary depending on health care setting, etiological agent, and associated comorbid conditions that are present. Medical history focusing on symptoms suggestive of CAP, associated complications, occurrence of comorbid conditions; and a thorough physical examination should be carried out.

Imaging Studies

In patients presenting with lower respiratory tract infection, presence of infiltrates on the chest radiograph suggests the diagnosis of CAP. Chest radiographs help in localizing the disease, defining disease extent and presence of complications.[2] Computed tomography is indicated in specific situations like excluding the presence of other diagnoses, when there is a suspicion of a fungal infection, when the chest radiograph is inconclusive, nonresolving/poorly resolving pneumonia, and for detection of complications.[2] Lung ultrasonography is increasingly being used for the diagnosis of pneumonia in adults and has been found to have high sensitivity (94%) and good specificity (96%).[9]

Laboratory Tests

Laboratory investigations are helpful in assessing the severity of CAP. These include complete hemogram, serum biochemistry, plasma glucose, and inflammatory markers, like C-reactive protein and procalcitonin, among others. In the initial assessment of patients with CAP, arterial oxygenation is important and is done by pulse oximetry or by arterial blood gas analysis. It is important to recognize hypoxemia early as it is associated with impending respiratory failure, need for ICU admission, and death.[10]

The diagnostic accuracy can be enhanced by ensuring adequate collection, transport, and microscopic screening for good quality sputum.[3,10-12] In severe CAP, other laboratory investigations, such as sputum staining, blood and sputum cultures, and urine testing for *Legionella* and pneumococcus antigens should be done. When pleural effusion is present a diagnostic thoracentesis should be done. Pleural fluid testing by aerobic and anaerobic cultures are indicated as presence of empyema which is associated with a poor prognosis.[10]

In patients with comorbid diseases and in patients seropositive for human immunodeficiency virus, blood culture and pleural fluid culture (when applicable) are helpful in ascertaining the etiological diagnosis as the incidence of bacteremia is high.[13]

Molecular Diagnostic Methods

With advancement in technology, molecular diagnostic methods are helpful in ascertaining the etiological cause and determining antibiotic susceptibility.[14]

Serological Tests

Serological tests are useful when atypical pathogens are suspected. Demonstration of a four-fold rise in the antibody titer in the convalescent specimen compared to acute-phase serum specimens is required for diagnosis.

Bronchoscopic Techniques

Bronchoscopic techniques are helpful in patients with HAP, as well as in patients with treatment failure, immunosuppression, and severe CAP. Common bronchoscopic techniques used include bronchoalveolar lavage (BAL) and protected specimen brushings (PSB). Demonstration of 104 colony forming units (CFU)/mL in BAL fluid samples and 103 CFU/mL in PSB samples is suggestive of infection.[15]

Diagnosis and Classification of Hospital-acquired and Ventilator-associated Pneumonia

Hospital-acquired pneumonia is defined as pneumonia acquired at 48 hours or more after hospital admission in nonventilated patients. It is suspected in patients who are hospitalized for 48 hours or more with a combination of (i) occurrence of a new or progressive lung infiltrates on chest X-ray, and (ii) presence of at least two of the followings: (a) fever more than or equal to 38°C, (b) leukocytosis or leukopenia, and (c) purulent secretions.

Ventilator-associated pneumonia is clinically diagnosed in patients who are receiving assisted mechanical ventilation and pneumonia develops in 48 hours or more after endotracheal intubation. Ventilator-associated pneumonia is diagnosed by the development of a new opacity on the chest X-ray and presence of two or more clinical features, including fever, leukopenia or leukocytosis, worsening hypoxemia, and purulent respiratory secretions.[5]

As a part of the initial evaluation, the American Thoracic Society (ATS)/ Infectious Disease Society of America (IDSA) guidelines recommend a chest X-ray, oxygenation status, blood cultures, and culture of the lower respiratory tract secretions obtained by invasive and noninvasive techniques obtained before initiation of antibiotic therapy.[10,11]

Microbiological Methods

Microbiological methods for the diagnosis of HAP include qualitative and quantitative analysis of the respiratory secretions. Common bronchoscopic techniques for HAP include BAL, PSB, and protected telescoping catheter (PTC). The presence of purulent respiratory secretions and positive culture qualitative, semiquantitative, or quantitative culture of sputum, endotracheal aspirate, BAL fluid, lung tissue, PSB or PTC are considered indicative of possible HAP/VAP.[15] Purulent secretions are defined as secretions from the lungs, bronchi, or trachea that contain more than 25 neutrophils and less than 10 squamous epithelial cells per low-power field.[15]

Blood cultures are indicated in patients suspected to have HAP/VAP as it has prognostic implications and positive blood cultures are more frequently associated with yield of MRSA.[16]

Assessment of Severity

The ATS and British Thoracic Society (BTS) guidelines for the management of patients with CAP recommend the use of severity scoring tools in conjunction with clinical assessment.[3,10,11]

Pneumonia severity index score

Pneumonia severity index (PSI) is a scoring system used to predict patients at risk of 30 day mortality.[17] Pneumonia severity index classifies the patents into five categories based on age, presence of comorbidities, physical examination, and laboratory data. Patients in classes I and II (score of ≤70) are treated as outpatients; patients in class III (score of 71–90) may benefit from brief hospitalization, while patients in classes IV and V (91 to >130) are generally admitted to the hospital.

CURB-65 score

CURB-65 score stratifies the patients based on the presence of confusion, urea levels, respiratory rate, blood pressure, and age 65 years or greater.[18] Patients with scores of 0–1 (low severity; corresponds to a 30 day mortality less than 3%), require an outpatient treatment. For a score of 2 (moderate severity; mortality of 9%), brief inpatient or supervised outpatient care is required. Urgent hospitalization is recommended for scores more than 3 (high severity; mortality of 15–40%). Patients with a score over 4 require ICU care.

SMART-COP score

The SMART-COP score (a mnemonic for systolic blood pressure, multilobar involvement on the chest radiograph, albumin level, respiratory rate, tachycardia, confusion, oxygenation, and arterial pH) identifies at risk patients who need additional evaluation/monitoring, even if not initially admitted to the ICU.[19]

Other severity criteria

The IDSA/ATS consensus guidelines on the management of CAP in adults have also been used to identify patients with severe CAP.[3] This scoring system comprises two major criteria and nine minor criteria. Severe CAP is defined as the presence of one of the two major criteria (i.e., the need for invasive mechanical ventilation or vasopressors) or three out of nine minor criteria (blood urea nitrogen level ≥20 mg/dL); confusion/disorientation; hypotension requiring aggressive fluid resuscitation; hypothermia (core temperature <36°C); leukopenia (total leucocyte count <4,000 cells/mm^3); multilobar infiltrates; ratio of arterial oxygen tension (PaO_2) to fraction of inspired oxygen (FiO_2) less than or equal to 250; respiratory rate greater than or equal to 30 breaths/min; thrombocytopenia (platelet count <100 × 10^3 cells/mm^3).

GUIDELINES FOR MANAGEMENT AND TREATMENT OF PNEUMONIA

Following diagnosis of pneumonia the clinician should decide the location for proper care and treatment. Patients at low-risk can be treated in the community as outpatient so that hospitalization and its consequences can be avoided.[3,10,11] The scoring systems described above can be used to decide as to which of the patients merit admission to the ICU and also help in predicting short-term mortality.[3,10,11,20]

Medical Management of Pneumonia

Outpatient Care

Severity scores helps clinicians to identify patients who may be appropriate for outpatient care, but the use of such scores must be interpreted after proper evaluation of patients. Outpatients with CAP should be advised to stop tobacco smoking, to take adequate rest, and to drink at least 1–2 L of fluids daily. The patient should also be advised to report any symptoms of chest pain, severe or increasing shortness of breath, or lethargy. Failure to improve within 48 hours should be a consideration for hospital admission. Up to 10% of outpatients do not respond to therapy and require hospitalization,[21] which increases the risk of infection with more virulent or resistant bacteria.[3] If the response to therapy is satisfactory, the patient should return within 10–14 days for repeat examination and a chest radiograph should be repeated one month after the episode of pneumonia.

Hospitalized Patients

Patients presenting with hypoxemia [arterial oxygen saturation measured by pulse oximetry (SpO_2) <90% or arterial oxygen tension (PaO_2) <60 mm Hg], or serious hemodynamic instability should be hospitalized regardless of their severity score. Hospitalized patients should receive appropriate oxygen therapy with the aim of maintaining SaO_2 at more than 92%. In patients with severe CAP and those requiring regular oxygen therapy, the parameters that are to be recorded and monitored at least twice daily or more frequently as required include mental status assessment, temperature, respirations, pulse, blood pressure, oxygen saturation, and inspired oxygen concentration. C-reactive protein is considered to be a sensitive marker of progression in CAP and should be periodically tested. A repeat chest X-ray is indicated in patients whose clinical improvement is not satisfactory.[11]

Intensive Care Unit Patients

Approximately, 10% of hospitalized patients with CAP require ICU admission. More recent severity scores (detailed above) should be used to predict ICU admission.[3,19,22] The concurrent occurrence of a numbers of risk factors has been observed to increase the likelihood of transfer to an ICU, need for vasopressors and assisted ventilation. These scoring systems also help in patients initially not admitted to ICU who are at-risk who will be requiring additional evaluation.

Antimicrobial Treatment of Community-acquired Pneumonia

Empirical Therapy

In general, the choice of empirical antibiotic treatment of CAP depends upon the disease severity and the presence of risk factors. Guidelines for the management of CAP have been published by various organizations, such as, IDSA/ATS and the British Thoracic Society (BTS).[3,11]

For Outpatient Treatment

The choice of antibiotic treatment for patients who are otherwise healthy who do not have risk factors for infection with drug-resistant organisms the initial choice of antibiotic includes either a macrolide (e.g., oral azithromycin 500 mg once daily followed by 250 mg once daily for duration of therapy) (IDSA/ATS strong recommendation, level I); or oral doxycycline (100 mg twice daily) (IDSA/ATS weak recommendation, level III).[3] If chronic comorbid conditions like diabetes mellitus, or underlying cardiac, pulmonary, hepatic, or renal disease is present or there is an immunocompromised state; there is a history of recent antibiotic use during the previous 3 months or in regions where there is a high rate of macrolide-resistant *Streptococcus pneumoniae*, a beta-lactam plus a macrolide (e.g., oral amoxicillin 1 g, three times daily plus azithromycin) is indicated (IDSA/ATS strong recommendation, level I).[3] Even though use of a respiratory fluoroquinolone (e.g., oral levofloxacin 750 mg once daily or oral moxifloxacin 400 mg once daily) has been recommended by the IDSA/ATS guidelines,[3] this is better avoided in countries like India where there is a high burden of tuberculosis (TB).

For Inpatient Treatment

For patients not in ICU, beta-lactam antibiotic, such as, cefotaxime, ceftriaxone, ampicillin, or ertapenem along with one of macrolides (IDSA/ATS strong recommendation, level I), or doxycycline (IDSA/ATS strong recommendation, Level III) are indicated.

For ICU patients, beta-lactam antibiotic like cefotaxime, ceftriaxone, or ampicillin-sulbactam along with either azithromycin (IDSA/ATS strong recommendation, level II) or a fluoroquinolone (IDSA/ATS strong recommendation, level I) are indicated. For patients who are allergic to penicillin, respiratory fluoroquinolone plus aztreonam can be used. As stated earlier, fluoroquinolones should be used with caution in the Indian setting where the prevalence of TB is high (Table 1).

For *Pseudomonas* infection, antipneumococcal, antipseudomonal beta-lactam (piperacillin/tazobactam, cefepime, imipenem, or meropenem) plus one of the following (IDSA/ATS moderate recommendation, level III), namely, ciprofloxacin, levofloxacin (750 mg dose); aminoglycoside plus azithromycin; aminoglycoside plus antipneumococcal fluoroquinolone are indicated. For patients who are penicillin allergic, aztreonam may be substituted for antipneumococcal, antipseudomonal beta-lactam. For community-acquired MRSA, vancomycin, linezolid, or (if susceptible) clindamycin are to be added (IDSA/ATS moderate recommendation, level III).

Empiric therapy for influenza should be initiated with a neuraminidase inhibitor in patients with compatible clinical syndrome during influenza season. In critically ill patients who require invasive mechanical ventilation, oseltamivir is preferred because zanamivir inhalation powder can clog ventilator tubing and has been associated with adverse events.[23,24] Early initiation of antiviral therapy (within 48 hours of symptom onset) is most efficacious;[25-29] however, all critically ill patients with suspected influenza should be treated empirically regardless of timing from symptom onset.

Table 1: Infectious Disease Society of America/American Thoracic Society Recommended Empirical Therapy for Severe Community-acquired Pneumonia[3]

- Beta-lactam (cefotaxime, ceftriaxone, or ampicillin/sulbactam) plus azithromycin or a respiratory fluoroquinolone
- For penicillin-allergic patients, a respiratory fluoroquinolone and aztreonam
- If *Pseudomonas* is a consideration, an antipneumococcal, antipseudomonal beta-lactam (piperacillin/tazobactam, cefepime, imipenem, or meropenem) plus either ciprofloxacin or levofloxacin (750 mg)

or

- Above beta-lactam plus an aminoglycoside and azithromycin

or

- Above beta-lactam plus an aminoglycoside and an antipneumococcal fluoroquinolone (for penicillin-allergic patients, substitute aztreonam for above beta-lactam)
- If CA-MRSA is considered, add vancomycin or linezolid

IDSA, Infectious Diseases Society of America; ATS, American Thoracic Society; CAP, community-acquired pneumonia; CA-MRSA, community-acquired methicillin-resistant *Staphylococcus aureus*.

Combination therapy

Combination therapy in severe CAP has been associated with improved outcomes in patients with bacteremic pneumococcal pneumonia, predominantly with macrolide-containing combination regimens.[30]

Pathogen-directed therapy

Once etiologic information becomes available from the microbiology laboratory, the empirical treatment should be modified to pathogen directed therapy. The narrowest spectrum agent should be used to prevent the development of antimicrobial resistance.

Nonresponse

Nonresponse is common in patients with CAP, occurring in 6–15% of hospitalized patients and approximately 40% of ICU patients.[31] Mortality rates are higher in nonresponders compared with responders.[31] The management of the nonresponding patient includes further diagnostic testing to identify the cause of pneumonia (if not determined on initial presentation), rule out the development of resistance on therapy, and to exclude complications such as empyema or nosocomial super-infection.

Duration of antibiotic treatment

Duration of therapy depends on disease severity, antimicrobial properties, patient immune status, and clinical response. Most patients with CAP receive 7–10 days of antimicrobial treatment, but little data or guidelines are available for critically ill patients who have traditionally received longer courses of therapy. Antimicrobial stewardship programs can help decrease duration and narrow the spectrum of antimicrobial therapy.[32]

Antimicrobial Treatment of Hospital-acquired and Ventilator-associated Pneumonia

In patients with nosocomial pneumonia (HAP and VAP) initial appropriate empiric antibiotic coverage should be based on the suspected pathogen in the appropriate clinical setting with institution of specific treatment once culture and drug-susceptibility data are available. In order to improve outcomes, guidelines[8] need to be adapted to the local microbiology to accurately predict pathogens, and help physicians to administer the most appropriate empiric antimicrobial therapy (Table 2).

Table 2: Recommended Initial Empiric Antibiotic Therapy for Hospital-acquired Pneumonia (Nonventilator-associated Pneumonia)

- If the patient is not at high risk of mortality and there are no factors predicting MRSA infection, one of the following:
  - Piperacillin-tazobactam 4.5 g IV q6h, or cefepime 2 g IV q8h, or levofloxacin 750 mg IV daily
  - Imipenem 500 mg IV q6h (meropenem 1 g IV q8h)
- If the patient is not at high risk of mortality, but with factors increasing the likelihood of MRSA, one of the following:
  - Piperacillin-tazobactam 4.5 g IV q6h, Or cefepime or ceftazidime 2 g IV q8h, or
  - Levofloxacin 750 mg IV daily (ciprofloxacin 400 mg IV q8h), or
  - Imipenem 500 mg IV q6h (meropenem 1 g IV q8h), or aztreonam 2 g IV q8h
  - Plus: Vancomycin (15 mg/kg IV q8–12h with a goal to target a trough level of 15–20 mg/mL

(A loading dose of 25–30 mg/kg may be administered for severe illness)

- High risk of mortality or receipt of intravenous antibiotics during the prior 90 days. Two of the following (avoid two beta-lactams):
  - Piperacillin-tazobactam 4.5 g IV q6h, or cefepime or ceftazidime 2 g IV q8h
  - Or, levofloxacin 750 mg IV daily (ciprofloxacin 400 mg IV q8h)
  - Or, imipenem 500 mg IV q6h (meropenem 1 g IV q8h)
  - Or, amikacin 15–20 mg/kg IV daily (gentamicin 5–7 mg/kg IV daily, tobramycin 5–7 mg/kg IV daily)
  - Plus: Vancomycin 15 mg/kg IV q8–12 h with a goal to target a trough level of 15–20 mg (a loading dose of 25–30 mg/kg may be administered for severe illness)
  - Or, linezolid 600 mg IV q12h

MRSA, methicillin-resistant *Staphylococcus aureus*; IV, intravenous.

Empirical Antibiotic Therapy

Empiric antibiotic regimen in nosocomial pneumonia should target *Staphylococcus aureus* and *Pseudomonas aeruginosa* and other gram-negative bacteria (IDSA/ATS strong recommendation/very low-quality evidence). The choice of antibiotic agent(s) is based on local epidemiology, severity of illness, and patient risk factors for MRSA infection. The risk factors for MRSA infection include intravenous antibiotic use in the preceding 90 days, hospitalization in a unit with more than 20% MRSA prevalence, or with unknown MRSA prevalence. The risk of mortality is high in patients with pneumonia requiring ventilatory support and those with septic shock. These details are shown in table 2.

Adjunctive inhaled antibiotic therapy as a treatment of last resort may be considered for patients who are not responding to intravenous antibiotics alone, whether the infecting organism is multidrug-resistant or not. If VAP is due to gram-negative bacilli that are susceptible to only aminoglycosides or polymyxins (colistin or polymyxin B), both inhaled and systemic antibiotics, rather than systemic antibiotics alone may be useful. Methicillin-resistant *Staphylococcus aureus* HAP/

VAP may be treated with vancomycin or linezolid rather than other antibiotics or antibiotic combinations. The choice between vancomycin and linezolid may be guided by patient-specific factors such as blood cell counts, concurrent prescriptions for serotonin reuptake inhibitors, renal function, and cost. In patients with HAP/VAP caused by a carbapenem-resistant pathogen that is sensitive only to polymyxins, IDSA recommends intravenous polymyxins (colistin or polymyxin B) and adjunctive inhaled colistin.

Treatment of Hospital-acquired Pneumonia/Ventilator-associated Pneumonia due to Pseudomonas aeruginosa

For patients with HAP/VAP due to *Pseudomonas aeruginosa*, IDSA/ATS guidelines recommend antibiotic choice for definitive therapy should be based on the results of antimicrobial susceptibility testing.[7,8] In setting with a high prevalence of extensively drug-resistant organisms, routine antimicrobial susceptibility testing should include sensitivity testing of *Pseudomonas aeruginosa* isolate to polymyxins (colistin or polymyxin B). Patients who are not in septic shock or at a high-risk for death, and for whom the results of antibiotic susceptibility testing are known, IDSA recommend monotherapy using an antibiotic to which the isolate is susceptible rather than combination therapy. For patients who are in septic shock or at high-risk of death and in whom antibiotic sensitivity is known combination therapy using two antibiotics to which the isolate is susceptible rather than monotherapy is advised.

Treatment of Hospital-acquired Pneumonia/Ventilator-associated Pneumonia due to Acinetobacter species

Patients with HAP/VAP caused by *Acinetobacter* spp., treatment with a carbapenem or ampicillin/sulbactam is indicated if the isolate is susceptible to these agents. If *Acinetobacter* spp. is sensitive only to polymyxins, intravenous polymyxin (colistin or polymyxin B) can be useful. In patients with HAP/VAP caused by *Acinetobacter* spp., is sensitive only to colistin, the IDSA/ATS guidelines recommend against the use of tigecycline (strong recommendation, low quality evidence) and adjunctive rifampicin (weak recommendation, moderate quality of evidence).[15,16]

Length of Therapy

For patients with VAP, IDSA/ATS recommend a 7 day course of antimicrobial therapy.[7,8] In certain situations, a shorter or longer duration of antibiotic treatment may be indicated, depending upon the rate of improvement of clinical, radiologic, and laboratory parameters. Further, for patients with HAP/VAP, IDSA/ATS guidelines recommend deescalated rather than fixed antibiotic therapy.[7,8]

COMPLICATIONS

Various complications can develop during the clinical course of pneumonia (Table 3) and these should be watched for and appropriate management must be instituted.

GUIDELINES FOR PREVENTION OF PNEUMONIA

Various preventive strategies, such as smoking cessation, avoiding alcohol consumption, maintaining good orodental hygiene, attention to good nutrition, among others are helpful in reducing the risk of CAP in adults.

In patients with HAP/VAP, nonpharmacological measures, such as hand washing and decontamination before and after contact with a patient should be practiced.[33,34] Specific hand washing agents, such as alcohol-based foams and lotions, may be more effective in hand disinfection compared to conventional use of soap and water.[35,36] Intubated patients should preferentially be kept in the semirecumbent position (30–45°) rather than supine (0°) to prevent aspiration, especially when receiving enteral feeding.[7,8,37] Tracheal intubation and reintubation increase the incidence of VAP by facilitating aspiration of bacteria.[37] Orotracheal intubation and orogastric tubes should be preferred compared to nasotracheal intubation and nasogastric tubes in order to prevent nosocomial sinusitis and to reduce the risk of VAP.[38] Continuous aspiration of subglottic secretions helps in reducing the risk of aspiration.[39] Maintenance of the endotracheal cuff pressure at approximately 20 cm H_2O may prevent leakage of bacterial pathogens around the cuff into the lower respiratory tract.[40]

Bacterial colonization of ventilator circuits occur rapidly.[37] Frequent changing of ventilator circuits has not been shown to reduce the incidence of VAP and must be avoided.[41] Continuous rotating beds in critically ill patients can reduce the occurrence of VAP.[42,43] Continuous lateral rotation therapy should be considered in patients at a higher risk of prolonged immobilization and respiratory infection.[34]

Table 3: Important Complications of Pneumonia

- Pleuropulmonary complications
  - Synpneumonic effusion
  - Parapneumonic effusion
  - Empyema
- Cardiovascular complications
  - New or worsening heart failure
  - New or worsening cardiac arrhythmia
  - Acute coronary syndromes
- Thromboembolic complications
  - Deep vein thrombosis
  - Pulmonary embolism
- Systemic complications
  - Bacteremia
  - Sepsis and related syndromes*

*Includes severe sepsis, septic shock, acute respiratory distress syndrome, acute kidney injury, multiple organ dysfunction syndrome etc.

International guidelines for the management of CAP recommend pneumococcal and influenza vaccination especially in risk population (young children, the elderly, patients with comorbidities, and the immunocompromised).[3,11,12]

CONCLUSION

Community-acquired pneumonia and HAP are important causes of mortality, morbidity and high costs globally. Disease severity scoring systems are helpful in deciding on hospitalization, need for ICU care and assessment of prognosis. New diagnostic methods for rapid clinical (e.g., lung ultrasound) and microbiological (e.g., molecular biological methods) diagnoses appear promising. Initiation of appropriate empirical antibiotic treatment is the cornerstone of management of patients with pneumonia. After the initiation of antibiotic treatment, management includes early shift to oral antibiotic treatment and stewardship as per the drug-susceptibility testing results.

Editor's Comment

Pneumonia is an important public health problem worldwide and is associated with a high mortality irrespective of the age groups involved. Early diagnosis and institution of therapy in the appropriate clinical setting are important steps to reduce health care costs and mortality. In most of the situations, an etiological diagnosis is either delayed or not achieved and hence, empirical antibiotic therapy is considered as the best approach to management. Another aspect of management is to establish the severity of pneumonia and selecting the appropriate settings for the treatment. This will considerably improve the outcome in pneumonia. Those who are nonresponders or delayed responders needs further diagnostic testing to identify the risk factors, etiology, antibiotic resistance, and complications such as empyema. Health care associated pneumonia and VAP raises further challenges to the clinician as the pneumonia is caused mostly by drug resistant organisms and patient has one or more other co morbidities. In spite of lot of information available on the subject, one often finds it difficult to make critical decisions. There are several evidence based guidelines to guide treatment decisions. It is important to frame evidence-based consensus guidelines for the management of pneumonia. This article lucidly describes the current practices in the management of pneumonia with reference to appropriate guidelines.

Ravindran Chetambath

REFERENCES

1. Kochanek KD, Murphy SL, Xu J, et al. Mortality in the United States, 2013. NCHS Data Brief. 2014;178:1-8.
2. Prina E, Ranzani OT, Torres A. Community-acquired pneumonia. *Lancet.* 2015;386:1097-108.
3. Wunderink RG, Anzueto A, Bartlett JG, et al. Infectious Diseases Society of America/American Thoracic Society consensus guidelines on the management of community acquired pneumonia in adults. *Clin Infect Dis.* 2007;44(Suppl. 2):S27-72.
4. Niederman MS, Bass JB Jr, Campbell GD, et al. Guidelines for the initial management of adults with community-acquired pneumonia: diagnosis, assessment of severity, and initial antimicrobial therapy. American Thoracic Society. Medical Section of the American Lung Association. *Am Rev Respir Dis.* 1993;148:1418-26.
5. Nair GB, Niederman MS. Nosocomial pneumonia: Lessons learned. *Crit Care Clin.* 2013;29:521-46.
6. Vincent JL, Rello J, Marshall J, et al. International study of the prevalence and outcomes of infection in intensive care units. *JAMA.* 2009;302:2323-29.
7. American Thoracic Society, Infectious Diseases Society of America. Guidelines for the management of adults with hospital-acquired, ventilator-associated, and healthcare associated pneumonia. *Am J Respir Crit Care Med.* 2005;171:388-416.
8. Kalil AC, Metersky ML, Klompas M, et al. Management of adults with hospital-acquired and ventilator-associated pneumonia: Clinical practice guidelines by the Infectious Diseases Society of America and the American Thoracic Society. *Clin Infect Dis.* 2016;63:e61-111.
9. Chastre J, Fagon JY. Ventilator-associated pneumonia. *Am J Respir Crit Care Med.* 2002;165:867-903.
10. Levin KP, Hanusa BH, Rotondi A, et al. Arterial blood gas and pulse oximetry in initial management of patients with community-acquired pneumonia. *J Gen Intern Med.* 2001;16(9):590-8.
11. Lim WS, Baudouin SV, George RC, et al. BTS guidelines for the management of community acquired pneumonia in adults: update 2009. *Thorax.* 2009;64(Suppl. 3):iii1-55.
12. Woodhead M, Blasi F, Ewig S, et al; Joint Taskforce of the European Respiratory Society and European Society for Clinical Microbiology and Infectious Diseases. Guidelines for the management of adult lower respiratory tract infections. *Clin Microbiol Infect.* 2011;17 (Suppl. 6):E1-59.
13. Cilloniz C, Torres A, Polverino E, et al. Community-acquired lung respiratory infections in HIV infected patients: microbial aetiology and outcome. *Eur Respir J.* 2014;43:1698-708.
14. Murdoch DR. Nucleic acid amplification tests for the diagnosis of pneumonia. *Clin Infect Dis.* 2003;36:1162-70.
15. Sirvent JM, Vidaur L, Gonzalez S, et al. Microscopic examination of intracellular organisms in protected bronchoalveolar mini-lavage fluid for the diagnosis of ventilator-associated pneumonia. *Chest.* 2003;123:518-23.
16. Rello J, Gallego M, Mariscal D, et al. The value of routine microbiologic investigation in the diagnosis of ventilator-associated pneumonia. *Am J Respir Crit Care Med.* 1997;156:196-200.
17. Aujesky D, Fine MJ. The pneumonia severity index: A decade after the initial derivation and validation. *Clin Infect Dis.* 2008;47(Suppl. 3):S133-9.
18. Lim WS, van der Eerden MM, Laing R, et al. Defining community acquired pneumonia severity on presentation to hospital: An international derivation and validation study. *Thorax.* 2003;58:377-82.
19. Charles PG, Wolfe R, Whitby M, et al. SMART-COP: A tool for predicting the need for intensive respiratory or vasopressor support in community-acquired pneumonia. *Clin Infect Dis.* 2008;47:375-84.
20. Chalmers JD, Singanayagam A, Hill AT. Predicting the need for mechanical ventilation and/or inotropic support for young adults admitted to the hospital with community-acquired pneumonia. *Clin Infect Dis.* 2008;47:1571-4.
21. Niederman M. In the clinic: Community-acquired pneumonia. *Ann Intern Med.* 2009;163(7):ITC1-17.
22. Capelastegui A, Gorordo I, Esteban C, et al. Development and validation of a clinical prediction rule for severe community-acquired pneumonia. *Am J Respir Crit Care Med.* 2006;174:1249-56.

23. Fiore AE, Fry A, Shay D, et al. Antiviral agents for the treatment and chemoprophylaxis of influenza—recommendations of the Advisory Committee on Immunization Practices (ACIP). *MMWR.* 2011;60:1-24.
24. Kiatboonsri S, Kiatboonsri C, Theerawit P. Fatal respiratory events caused by zanamivir nebulization. *Clin Infect Dis.* 2010;50:620-24.
25. Nicholson KG, Aoki FY, Osterhaus AD, et al. Efficacy and safety of oseltamivir in treatment of acute influenza: A randomised controlled trial. Neuraminidase Inhibitor Flu Treatment Investigator Group. *Lancet.* 2000;355:1845-50.
26. Kaiser L, Wat C, Mills T, et al. Impact of oseltamivir treatment on influenza related lower respiratory tract complications and hospitalizations. *Arch Intern Med.* 2003;163:1667-72.
27. Jefferson T, Demicheli V, Rivetti D, et al. Antivirals for influenza in healthy adults: Systematic review. *Lancet.* 2006;367:303-13.
28. Rodríguez A, Díaz E, Martín-Loeches I, et al. Impact of early oseltamivir treatment on outcome in critically ill patients with 2009 pandemic influenza A. *J Antimicrob Chemother.* 2011;66:1140-9.
29. Kumar A. Early versus late oseltamivir treatment in severely ill patients with 2009 pandemic influenza A (H1N1): Speed is life. *J Antimicrob Chemother.* 2011;66:959-63.
30. Asadi L, Sligl WI, Eurich DT, et al. Macrolide-based regimens and mortality in hospitalized patients with community-acquired pneumonia: A systematic review and meta-analysis. *Clin Infect Dis.* 2012;55:371-80.
31. Rosón B, Carratalà J, Fernández-Sabé N, et al. Causes and factors associated with early failure in hospitalized patients with community-acquired pneumonia. *Arch Intern Med.* 2004;164:502-8.
32. Avdic E, Cushinotto LA, Hughes AH, et al. Impact of an antimicrobial stewardship intervention on shortening the duration of therapy for community-acquired pneumonia. *Clin Infect Dis.* 2012;54:1581-87.
33. Iregui MG, Vaughan WM, Kollef MH. Nonpharmacological prevention of hospital-acquired pneumonia. *Semin Respir Crit Care Med.* 2002;23:489-96.
34. Klein BS, Perloff WH, Maki DG. Reduction of nosocomial infection during pediatric intensive care by protective isolation. *N Engl J Med.* 1989;320:1714-21.
35. Girou E, Loyeau S, Legrand P, et al. Efficacy of hand rubbing with alcohol based solution versus standard hand washing with antiseptic soap: randomized clinical trial. *BMJ.* 2002;325:362-68.
36. Kampf G, Jarosch R, Ruden H. Effectiveness of alcoholic hand disinfectants against methicillin resistant Staphylococcus aureus. *Chirurg.* 1997;68:264-68.
37. Torres A, Ewig S, Lode H, et al. Defining, treating and preventing hospital acquired pneumonia: European perspective. *Intensive Care Med.* 2009;35:9-29.
38. Rouby JJ, Laurent P, Gosnach M, et al. Risk factors and clinical relevance of nosocomial maxillary sinisitis in the critically ill. *Am J Respir Crit Care Med.* 1994;150:776-83.
39. Kollef MH, Skubas NJ, Sundt TM. A randomized clinical trial of continuous aspiration of subglottic secretions in cardiac surgery patients. *Chest.* 1999;116:1339-46.
40. Cook D, De Jonghe B, Brochard L, et al. Influence of airway management on ventilator-associated pneumonia: Evidence from randomized trials. *JAMA.* 1998;279:781-87.
41. Dreyfuss D, Djedaini K, Weber P, et al. Prospective study of nosocomial pneumonia and of patient and circuit colonization during mechanical ventilation with circuit changes every 48 hours versus no change. *Am Rev Respir Dis.* 1991;143:738-43.
42. Fink MP, Helsmoortel CM, Stein KL, et al. The efficacy of an oscillating bed in the prevention of lower respiratory tract infection in critically ill victims of blunt trauma. A prospective study. *Chest.* 1990;97:132-7.
43. Gentilello L, Thompson DA, Tonnesen AS, et al. Effect of a rotating bed on the incidence of pulmonary complications in critically ill patients. *Crit Care Med.* 1988;16:783-6.

World Clin Pulm Crit Care Med. 2019;6(1):76-87.

Community-acquired Pneumonia

[1]Aditya Jindal DNB DM, [2,*]Surinder K Jindal MD FCCP FAMS FNCCP

[1]Jindals Clinics, Chandigarh, India
[2]Department of Pulmonary Medicine, Post Graduate Institute of Medical Education and Research Chandigarh, India

ABSTRACT

Community-acquired pneumonia (CAP) is one of the most common infections in humans; it is common across all age groups and does not have any gender predilection. As a disease syndrome, CAP is one of the oldest known to us, historically. It has been associated with significant morbidity and mortality throughout the ages. Although, the discovery of antibiotics and vaccination have been major steps in the fight against CAP, the emergence of drug resistance pathogens and newer at risk populations means that the war is still not over. This is especially relevant to countries in the developing world, where the incidence of drug resistance is extremely high, in addition to the already high prevalence of CAP.

INTRODUCTION

According to the joint Indian Chest Society and the National College of Chest Physicians guidelines on community and hospital-acquired pneumonia, CAP can be defined based on clinical and/or radiographic findings. In the absence of chest radiograph, CAP is defined as: (i) symptoms of an acute lower respiratory tract illness (cough with or without expectoration, shortness of breath, pleuritic chest pain) for less than 1 week; (ii) at least one systemic feature (temperature >37.7°C, chills, rigors, and/or severe malaise); (iii) new signs on chest examination (bronchial breath sounds and/or crackles); and (iv) no other explanation for the illness.

With the availability of a chest radiograph, CAP is defined as symptoms and signs as above with evidence of new radiological shadows for which there is no alternative explanation (e.g., not due to pulmonary edema or infarction). Radiological shadows which may be seen are lobar or patchy consolidation,

*Corresponding author
Email: dr.skjindal@gmail.com

interstitial opacities, loss of a normal diaphragmatic, cardiac or mediastinal silhouette, or bilateral perihilar opacities, without any other obvious cause.[1]

EPIDEMIOLOGY

The incidence of CAP varies widely from country to country and at different ages; it is generally more common at extremes of age. The incidence rate in adults are roughly 2.5 per 1,000 populations in the United States of America (USA) and rise with increasing age. Approximately 1.1 million people had to be hospitalized while 50,000 deaths occurred.

Though studies and data from the developing world are fragmentary, some data are available. In India, the number of deaths due to lower respiratory tract infections was 35.1/100,000 populations in 2008, accounting for approximately 20% of mortality due to infectious diseases.[2,3]

Community-acquired pneumonia is more common in malnourished population, overcrowded localities, and in persons with a low socioeconomic status. Use of alcohol, chronic smoking, and drug abuse all predispose to the development of CAP. The presence of chronic disease states like diabetes mellitus, renal failure, and chronic cardiovascular and pulmonary disorders also predispose to develop pneumonia. Of importance is the group of immunocompromised individuals, who are extremely prone to develop this syndrome. The number of persons in this group is constantly increasing, due to the pandemic of human immunodeficiency virus/acquired immunodeficiency syndrome (HIV/AIDS), progressive use of immunosuppressive therapies and the development of transplantation.[4]

ETIOLOGY

In the pre-antibiotic era, *Streptococcus pneumoniae* or the pneumococcus caused more than 90% of cases of CAP. In present times, it is still the most common cause of CAP worldwide, with incidence rates varying from one-fourth to one-third of all pneumonias. However, as the microbiological diagnosis of CAP is difficult to determine in 40–70% of cases, this estimate may be fallacious. The incidence of pneumococcal pneumonia has been coming down in recent years in the developed world—especially in the United States—because of the widespread use of pediatric and adult immunization as well as the decreased incidence of smoking. In the developing world, this may not hold true.

Other bacteria which are important causes of CAP include *Haemophilus influenzae, Staphylococcus aureus, Pseudomonas aeruginosa*, or other gram-negative rods, *Moraxella catarrhalis*, mixed microaerophilic, and anaerobic oral flora. *Mycoplasma pneumoniae, Chlamydophila pneumonia*, and *Legionella pneumophila* are important causes of the atypical pneumonias, where there is discordance between mild symptomatology and alarming radiological findings. *Staphylococcus* and *Pseudomonas* species are important pathogens in patients who have underlying chronic obstructive pulmonary disease or bronchiectasis.[2,4-8]

Viral infections are also important causes of CAP. Influenza viruses are the most common pathogens and may be responsible for one-third to half of all pneumonia cases during epidemics. The most famous pandemic of influenza was just after World War I, known as the "Spanish flu," which was responsible for millions of deaths worldwide. In fact, according to some estimates, 7% of the population in some parts of India died during this time. A recent pandemic occurred in 2009, characterized by severe acute respiratory distress syndrome (ARDS), high morbidity and mortality (acute respiratory distress syndrome). Other viruses causing CAP include parainfluenza virus, respiratory syncytial virus, adenovirus, human metapneumovirus, coronavirus, and rhinovirus.[9,10]

Depending upon the geographical area some causes are more common. *Coxiella burnetii* and histoplasmosis are common in some parts of the United States while *Pencillium marneffei* is common in South East Asia. Patients with HIV/AIDS and other immunosuppressed individuals are predisposed to certain unusual infections in addition to the common ones. These include *Pneumocystis jirovecii*, *Aspergillus* species, *Candida* species, *Nocardia* species, and mucormycosis.

CLINICAL PRESENTATION

The symptomatology of CAP varies based on the extent of involvement of the lungs, immune status, systemic dissemination, and other factors. Classical or typical pneumonia presents as an acute onset illness with high grade fever, productive cough, breathlessness, pleuritic chest pain, malaise, and fatigue. Clinical examination reveals the presence of tachycardia, tachypnea, and fever. Hypotension and low oxygen saturation, if present, denote severe pneumonia and sepsis. Chest examination may show the presence of dullness on percussion, bronchial breathing, and coarse crackles. Atypical pneumonia, generally caused by microorganisms such as Chlamydia, *Mycoplasma, Legionella*, respiratory viruses, and others presents in a less acute manner. Patients have more of symptoms such as malaise and fatigue and the syndrome may be preceded by an upper respiratory tract infection. However, the distinction between these two types is not absolute and only serves as a rough guide at best.

The frequency of these symptoms is variable and they may occur in different combinations. Some etiologies like Legionella pneumonia, Q fever, etc. may be associated with specific signs and symptoms. No combination of symptoms is enough to distinguish one cause from another. Also, elderly and immunocompromised individuals may report less symptoms as compared to the severity of illness. Severe infections may precipitate the development of ARDS, which is associated with additional morbidity and mortality. It should be kept in mind that severity in CAP varies widely, with mild illnesses requiring only outpatient therapy to severe disease leading to prolonged mechanical ventilation.

DIAGNOSIS

The diagnosis of CAP is based primarily on a high degree of suspicion, supplemented by radiological and microbiological investigations. Clinical features may point to the diagnosis with varying sensitivity and specificity.

Radiological Investigations

The chest X-ray has been said to be the cornerstone of the diagnostic protocol. However, as with any investigation, the sensitivity and specificity should be kept in mind before treating the X-ray report as final. The following findings may be present on the chest radiograph: (i) focal lung opacification with air bronchograms, (ii) presence of the silhouette sign, (iii) an area of increased opacity bounded by a well-defined interface against adjacent aerated lung, (iv) increased attenuation of the cardiac shadow, and (v) asymmetric or multifocal distribution of opacities. The X-ray may also show the presence of complications like pleural effusions, empyema, and infiltrates suggestive of ARDS.[11]

Computed tomography (CT) scans are more precise for the diagnosis of CAP compared to chest radiographs. The findings on CT is suggestive of CAP that include lobar or multifocal consolidation, air bronchograms, and centrilobular nodules. Computed tomography is also helpful in the assessment of complications and for the differential diagnosis. However, CT is an expensive investigation with significant radiation exposure and the vast majority of patients do not need it. Its use in the diagnostic algorithm of CAP is mainly limited to the above mentioned indications, viz., assessment of complications, differential diagnosis, and/or for cases with atypical symptoms.

In recent years, lung ultrasound has been explored as an alternative to conventional radiological techniques in the diagnosis of community-acquired pneumonia. Besides the obvious advantage of being free from radiation, ultrasound also has the advantage of being immediately available, also it can be done at the bedside or in the outpatient department. The sensitivity and specificity is said to be better than conventional chest radiography. However, lung ultrasonography has some disadvantages too—it is significantly observer dependent, it might not pick up certain complications or differential diagnosis and may require extra regulatory approval, especially in the Indian context.[12,13]

In conclusion, it may be said most patients with mild infections would not need any radiological investigations, while the investigational flowchart would start with the chest X-ray in the rest.

Microbiological Investigations

Again, many patients who have mild infections may not require investigation. However, in patients who are immunocompromised or are hospitalized or severely ill, an effort should be made to identify etiological agent. Sputum culture and Gram stain are the basic investigations to be done, though the sample should be acceptable. The sensitivity and specificity varies widely. In the Indian context sputum examination for acid-fast bacilli is a must because of the high prevalence of tuberculosis.

Blood cultures have low sensitivity but high specificity in identifying the etiology. They should be done in all hospitalized and seriously ill patients. Immunocompromised patients may have a higher yield of culture positivity.

Molecular techniques have recently come to the fore. However, the sensitivity, specificity, and positive and negative predictive value for these tests have not been established in developing countries. These should be done only in specific clinical situations till further data becomes available. Reverse transcriptase polymerase chain reaction for influenza testing is better established but should be done only in case of epidemics or in certain situations.[1,3,14]

Biomarkers

The role of biomarkers in the diagnosis of CAP is still under investigation. Conceptually, the use of a single test that could determine the diagnosis is attractive. However, the practical utility has not yet been established. The two biomarkers which have been most extensively studied are procalcitonin and C-reactive protein. Both of them have shown some promise, especially when measured serially. Although, procalcitonin seems to be of use as an adjunct to other diagnostic methods, the routine use of these biomarkers is still not recommended.[15-17]

TREATMENT

Community-acquired pneumonia has a wide spectrum of clinical presentation and severity. Some of the severe forms of CAP have high mortality risks varying from 10 to 30% or more. The management recommendations will also depend upon the decision regarding the site of care for a particular patient. The treatment of CAP can be discussed under two broad categories—antimicrobial therapy and supportive therapy. The choice of antibiotics and other supportive therapy however, is determined by the disease severity, presence of respiratory failure, and other complications. A patient with an increased risk of failure needs admission in the wards or in the intensive care unit depending upon the degree of severity or clinical instability. Admission for mild cases is avoidable to save in-patient costs and prevent other hospital-acquired complications. The management principles therefore, tend to differ with the risk classification and severity scores.

Severity Scoring

Several severity scores are available for purposes of quantification of risk development. The most commonly employed scores include the following:
1. Pneumonia severity index (PSI)
2. CURB-65
3. CRB-65
4. SMART-COP
5. SMRT-CO
6. A-DROP
7. Others.

The most extensively validated are the PSI, CRB-65 or CURB-65, and SMART-COP. CURB-65 is among the most commonly used scores as it is validated and also easy to use in a busy clinical setting. Points are given to six separate measurements [confusion, urea >7 nmol/L, respiratory rate >30/min, low blood pressure (diastolic blood pressure <60 mm Hg or systolic blood pressure <90 mm Hg), age >65 years, with a range from 0-5]. Based on this score, patients can be stratified according to increasing risk of mortality, ranging from 0.7% (score 0) to 40% (score 4). A model based only on clinical features (confusion, respiratory rate, blood pressure and age; CRB-65 score) was also found to correlate well with risk of mortality and need for mechanical ventilation. In addition, the use of low oxygen saturation has also been shown to be associated with increased mortality and is an independent marker of worse prognosis.[3,8-25]

Antibiotic Treatment

Initial empirical antibiotic treatment is based on factors such as the most likely pathogen(s); local susceptibility patterns; pharmacokinetics/pharmacodynamics of antibiotics; and compliance, safety, and cost of the drugs to be used. Empirical therapy is primarily aimed at *Streptococcus pneumoniae* as the most frequent organism causing CAP. The commonly used antibiotics are either beta-lactams or macrolides in the outpatient setting.[1,3,14]

Streptococcus pneumoniae is also the most common cause of severe CAP. So, therapy of inpatients should also be directed toward covering this organism. However, inpatients who have severe CAP might have resistant or other pathogens; hence, the antibiotic coverage might have to be modified. Immunocompromised patients are prone to a wide variety of microorganisms; the empirical antibiotics should cover these organisms too (Table 1). The use of fluoroquinolones should be restricted in areas of high prevalence of tuberculosis as indiscriminate use of these drugs may lead to drug resistance and also partial treatment of tuberculosis with masking of symptoms. These drugs should be given in CAP only after the treating physician is satisfied that the disease is not due to tuberculosis.[1,26,27]

In patients having severe disease or immunocompromised state, combination antibiotic treatment may be used. Monotherapy suffices in less serious cases. Combination therapy has been shown to reduce the mortality in multiple studies.

The time of first dose of antibiotics has been found to be critical, especially in severe CAP. In this situation, the aim should be to given the first dose within the first hour of admission. However, in outpatients, efforts should be made to establish the diagnosis before starting the treatment. The treatment duration for outpatients is generally 3–5 days; while for inpatients the duration may be extended to 5–7 days. In patients with complications such as empyemas, endocarditis, meningitis, etc. the treatment duration needs to be longer. However, most patients can be treated with shorter courses of antibiotics. The doses of common drugs used are given in table 2.[28-32]

Adjunctive Therapies

In addition to supportive management of patients, various additive therapies have been tried from time to time. The most widely studied of these therapies is the

Table 1: Empirical Treatment of Community-acquired Pneumonia

Outpatients	Azithromycin, fluoroquinolones, amoxicillin, co-amoxiclav
Inpatients	Amoxicillin, co-amoxiclav, ceftriaxone, cefepime, cefoperazone-sulbactam, imipenem, meropenem
For staphylococcal coverage	Vancomycin, linezolid, clindamycin
For pseudomonas coverage	Piperacillin-tazobactam, ceftazidime, meropenem, imipenem
Influenza	Oseltamivir, zanamivir

Table 2: Common Drugs and Dosages Used in Community-acquired Pneumonia

Amoxicillin	0.5–1 g thrice daily (PO or IV)
Co-amoxiclav	625 mg thrice a day to 1 g twice daily (PO)/1.2 g thrice daily (IV)
Azithromycin	500 mg daily (PO or IV)
Ceftriaxone	1–2 g twice daily (IV)
Piperacillin–tazobactam	4.5 g four times a day (IV)
Imipenem	0.5–1 g three to four times a day (IV)
Meropenem	1 g thrice daily (IV)

IV, intravenous; PO, per os.

use of adjunctive corticosteroids. Multiple authors have argued for and against the use of steroids in CAP. The overall consensus is that steroids should not be used in routine cases, though use in specific situations may be useful. Other therapies such as activated protein C, immunoglobulin, anticoagulants, antiplatelet drugs, granulocyte-colony-stimulating factor, statins, probiotics, chest physiotherapy, β2-agonists, inhaled nitric oxide, etc. have not been found to be useful.[33-41]

Severe pneumonia going into ARDS requires the use of mechanical ventilation according to the ARDS net strategy. This involves use of low tidal volumes, positive end-expiratory pressure, permissive hypercapnia, etc. Influenza infections, especially during pandemics, lead to very severe ARDS and patients often require prolonged mechanical ventilation. Other complications of CAP also need to be treated accordingly. Empyema need to be drained by either intercostal chest tubes or pigtails and may occasionally require surgery. Endocarditis, meningitis, pus collections in other organ, etc. may be present and need to be handled properly.

Vaccination

There are at present vaccines for two pathogens available to prevent CAP. The first pathogen is *Streptococcus pneumoniae*, for which two vaccines are available. One is the older 23 valent polysaccharide antigen vaccine while the other is the protein polysaccharide conjugate vaccine which covers 13 serotypes. While both have their advantages and disadvantages, they are recommended to be given in series in high-risk individuals and in healthy adults more than 65 years of age. These vaccines prevent against both invasive and noninvasive pneumococcal pneumonia.[42]

Vaccines are also available for influenza virus infections. These include live, inactivated, recombinant, and high dose variants. Some countries recommend the use of these vaccines annually for the entire population.

In India, the vaccine is recommended for pregnant females, heath care workers, and other high-risk groups. Vaccines for other respiratory pathogens are being developed and may see the light of the day soon.[6,43-51] High-risk groups where these vaccines are recommended are mentioned in table 3.

Table 3: High-risk Groups for Community-acquired Pneumonia

Pneumococcal disease	Influenza
• Chronic cardiovascular disease • Pulmonary, renal, or liver disease • Diabetes mellitus • Cerebrospinal fluid leaks • Alcoholism • Asplenia • Immunocompromised states	• Chronic cardiovascular or pulmonary disease (including asthma) • Chronic metabolic disease (including diabetes mellitus) • Renal failure • Hemoglobinopathies • Immunocompromised states • Compromised airway or increased aspiration risk

CONCLUSION

Community-acquired pneumonia is a serious health problem worldwide, both historically and in the present scenario. The spread of the HIV/AIDS pandemic and the use of immunosuppressive medications have put new populations at risk of developing CAP. The diagnosis depends on clinical acumen and supportive investigations. Treatment should be started early and severe cases should be triaged to the intensive care unit for appropriate management. The development of new vaccines and drugs might hold hope for the future.

Editor's Comment

The morbidity and mortality of community-acquired pneumonia remains high despite the availability of newer and more potent antibiotics along with improved facilities for supportive care. An increasing number of patients with community-acquired pneumonia who are either on immunomodulatory therapy or immuno-compromised have made the management of community-acquired pneumonia all the more challenging. The spectrum of pathogens involved in causing pneumonia in these individuals, the varying clinical presentations and difficulty in diagnosis are much worrying. The new and emerging pathogens, especially the viruses, are causing pneumonia worldwide in epidemic proportions. There are many objective tools like PSI and CURB-65 to assess the severity, and these should be used in day to day practice to take evidence based management decisions. CRB-65 can be easily used in the outpatient departments, and site of care decisions can be made based on such validated tools in association with clinical judgment. Empirical antibiotic choice should be based on recommendations, as data have not shown any improvement with the use of higher antibiotics. Use of newer antibiotics and higher spectrum antibiotics are on the rise and is a global concern. A rational use of antibiotics based on the prevalent organisms and local sensitivity pattern should be done. Effort should be made to identify the pathogen and tailor antibiotic use accordingly. This will help in improving the outcome and decreasing the emergence of drug resistance. Authors have brought out answers to all the pertinent questions a physician may raise with regard to community-acquired pneumonia.

Ravindran Chetambath

REFERENCES

1. Gupta D, Agarwal R, Aggarwal AN, et al. Guidelines for diagnosis and management of community- and hospital-acquired pneumonia in adults: Joint ICS/NCCP(I) recommendations. *Lung India.* 2012;29 (Suppl 2):S27-62.
2. Aston SJ. Pneumonia in the developing world: Characteristic features and approach to management. Respirology (Carlton, Vic). 2017;22(7):1276-87.
3. Mandell LA, Wunderink RG, Anzueto A, et al. Infectious Diseases Society of America/American Thoracic Society consensus guidelines on the management of community-acquired pneumonia in adults. *Clin Infect Dis.* 2007;44 (Suppl 2):S27-72.
4. Musher DM, Thorner AR. Community acquired pneumonia. *N Engl J Med.* 2014;371:1619-28.
5. Ansarie M, Kasmani A. Community acquired pneumonia in Pakistan: An analysis on the literature published between 2003 and 2013. *J Pak Med Assoc.* 2014;64(12):1405-9.
6. DeAntonio R, Yarzabal JP, Cruz JP, et al. Epidemiology of community-acquired pneumonia and implications for vaccination of children living in developing and newly industrialized countries: A systematic literature review. *Hum Vaccin Immunother.* 2016;12(9):2422-40.
7. Marchello C, Dale AP, Thai TN, et al. Prevalence of atypical pathogens in patients with cough and community-acquired pneumonia: A meta-analysis. *Ann Fam Med.* 2016;14(6):552-66.
8. Sharma L, Losier A, Tolbert T, et al. Atypical pneumonia: Updates on Legionella, Chlamydophila, and Mycoplasma pneumonia. *Clin Chest Med.* 2017;38(1):45-58.
9. Burk M, El-Kersh K, Saad M, et al. Viral infection in community-acquired pneumonia: a systematic review and meta-analysis. *Eur Respir Rev.* 2016;25(140):178-88.
10. Galvan JM, Rajas O, Aspa J. Review of non-bacterial infections in respiratory medicine: Viral pneumonia. *Arch Bronconeumol.* 2015;51(11):590-7.
11. Andronikou S, Lambert E, Halton J, et al. Guidelines for the use of chest radiographs in community-acquired pneumonia in children and adolescents. *Pediatric Radiol.* 2017;47(11):1405-11.
12. Stadler JAM, Andronikou S, Zar HJ. Lung ultrasound for the diagnosis of community-acquired pneumonia in children. *Pediatr Radiol.* 2017;47(11):1412-9.
13. Ye X, Xiao H, Chen B, et al. Accuracy of lung ultrasonography versus chest radiography for the diagnosis of adult community-acquired pneumonia: Review of the literature and meta-analysis. *PloS One.* 2015;10(6): e0130066.
14. Levy ML, Le Jeune I, Woodhead MA, et al. Primary care summary of the British Thoracic Society guidelines for the management of community acquired pneumonia in adults: 2009 update. Endorsed by the Royal College of General Practitioners and the Primary Care Respiratory Society UK. *Prim Care Respir J.* 2010;19(1):21-7.
15. Shaddock EJ. How and when to use common biomarkers in community-acquired pneumonia. *Pneumonia (Nathan Qld).* 2016;8:17.
16. Tang H, Huang T, Jing J, et al. Effect of procalcitonin-guided treatment in patients with infections: A systematic review and meta-analysis. *Infection.* 2009;37(6):497-507.
17. Schuetz P, Chiappa V, Briel M, et al. Procalcitonin algorithms for antibiotic therapy decisions: a systematic review of randomized controlled trials and recommendations for clinical algorithms. *Arch Intern Med.* 2011;171(15):1322-31.
18. Falcone M, Corrao S, Venditti M, et al. Performance of PSI, CURB-65, and SCAP scores in predicting the outcome of patients with community-acquired and healthcare-associated pneumonia. *Intern Emerg Med.* 2011;6(5):431-6.
19. Heppner HJ, Sehlhoff B, Niklaus D, et al. [Pneumonia Severity Index (PSI), CURB-65, and mortality in hospitalized elderly patients with aspiration pneumonia]. *Z Gerontol Geriatr.* 2011;44(4):229-34.
20. Ananda-Rajah MR, Charles PG, Melvani S, et al. Comparing the pneumonia severity index with CURB-65 in patients admitted with community acquired pneumonia. *Scand J Infect Dis.* 2008;40(4):293-300.

21. Huaman MA, Diaz-Kuan A, Hegab S, et al. CURB-65 and SMRT-CO in the prediction of early transfers to the intensive care unit among patients with community-acquired pneumonia initially admitted to a general ward. *J Hosp Med.* 2011;6(9):513-8.
22. Myint PK, Sankaran P, Musonda P, et al. Performance of CURB-65 and CURB-age in community-acquired pneumonia. *Int J Clin Pract.* 2009;63(9):1345-50.
23. Parsonage M, Nathwani D, Davey P, et al. Evaluation of the performance of CURB-65 with increasing age. *Clin Microbiol Infect.* 2009;15(9):858-64.
24. Shah BA, Ahmed W, Dhobi GN, et al. Validity of pneumonia severity index and CURB-65 severity scoring systems in community acquired pneumonia in an Indian setting. *Indian J Chest Dis Allied Sci.* 2010;52(1): 9-17.
25. Usui K, Tanaka Y, Noda H, et al. [Comparison of three prediction rules for prognosis in community acquired pneumonia: Pneumonia Severity Index (PSI), CURB-65, and A-DROP]. *Nihon Kokyuki Gakkai Zasshi.* 2009; 47(9):781-5.
26. Chang KC, Leung CC, Yew WW, et al. Newer fluoroquinolones for treating respiratory infection: do they mask tuberculosis? *Eur Respir J.* 2010;35(3):606-13.
27. Chen TC, Lu PL, Lin CY,et al. Fluoroquinolones are associated with delayed treatment and resistance in tuberculosis: A systematic review and meta-analysis. *Int J Infect Dis.* 2011;15(3):e211-6.
28. Horita N, Otsuka T, Haranaga S, et al. Beta-lactam plus macrolides or beta-lactam alone for community-acquired pneumonia: A systematic review and meta-analysis. *Respirology (Carlton, Vic).* 2016;21(7):1193-200.
29. Mantero M, Tarsia P, Gramegna A, et al. Antibiotic therapy, supportive treatment and management of immunomodulation-inflammation response in community acquired pneumonia: Review of recommendations. *Multidiscip Respir Med.* 2017;12:26.
30. Phua J, Dean NC, Guo Q, et al. Severe community-acquired pneumonia: Timely management measures in the first 24 hours. *Crit Care.* 2016;20:237.
31. Pletz MW, Rohde GG, Welte T, et al. Advances in the prevention, management, and treatment of community-acquired pneumonia. *F1000Res.* 2016;5.
32. Prina E, Ceccato A, Torres A. New aspects in the management of pneumonia. Crit Care. 2016;20(1):267.
33. Bi J, Yang J, Wang Y, et al. Efficacy and safety of adjunctive corticosteroids therapy for severe community-acquired pneumonia in adults: An updated systematic review and meta-analysis. *PloS One.* 2016;11(11):e0165942.
34. Feldman C, Anderson R. Corticosteroids in the adjunctive therapy of community-acquired pneumonia: An appraisal of recent meta-analyses of clinical trials. *J Thorac Dis.* 2016;8(3):E162-71.
35. Annane D, Bellissant E, Bollaert PE, et al. Corticosteroids in the treatment of severe sepsis and septic shock in adults: a systematic review. *JAMA.* 2009;301(22):2362-75.
36. Chen Y, Li K, Pu H, et al. Corticosteroids for pneumonia. *Cochrane Database Syst Rev.* 2011(3):CD007720.
37. Maes ML, Fixen DR, Linnebur SA. Adverse effects of proton-pump inhibitor use in older adults: A review of the evidence. *Ther Adv Drug Saf.* 2017;8(9):273-97.
38. Mikami K, Suzuki M, Kitagawa H, et al. Efficacy of corticosteroids in the treatment of community-acquired pneumonia requiring hospitalization. *Lung.* 2007;185(5):249-55.
39. Salluh JI, Povoa P, Soares M, et al. The role of corticosteroids in severe community-acquired pneumonia: A systematic review. *Crit Care.* 2008;12(3):R76.
40. Salluh JI, Soares M, Coelho LM, et al. Impact of systemic corticosteroids on the clinical course and outcomes of patients with severe community-acquired pneumonia: A cohort study. *J Crit Care.* 2011;26(2):193-200.
41. Tang BM, Craig JC, Eslick GD, et al. Use of corticosteroids in acute lung injury and acute respiratory distress syndrome: A systematic review and meta-analysis. *Crit Care Med.* 2009;37(5):1594-603.
42. Bonten MJ, Huijts SM, Bolkenbaas M, et al. Polysaccharide conjugate vaccine against pneumococcal pneumonia in adults. *N Engl J Med.* 2015;372(12):1114-25.

43. Tin Tin Htar M, Stuurman AL, Ferreira G, et al. Effectiveness of pneumococcal vaccines in preventing pneumonia in adults, a systematic review and meta-analyses of observational studies. *PloS One.* 2017;12(5): e0177985.
44. Campitelli MA, Rosella LC, Stukel TA, et al. Influenza vaccination and all-cause mortality in community-dwelling elderly in Ontario, Canada, a cohort study. *Vaccine.* 2010;29(2):240-6.
45. Christenson B, Pauksen K, Sylvan SP. Effect of influenza and pneumococcal vaccines in elderly persons in years of low influenza activity. *Virol J.* 2008;5:52.
46. Huss A, Scott P, Stuck AE, et al. Efficacy of pneumococcal vaccination in adults: A meta-analysis. *CMAJ.* 2009;180(1):48-58.
47. Expert Group of the Association of Physicians of India on Adult Immunization in India. The Association of Physicians of India evidence-based clinical practice guidelines on adult immunization. *J Assoc Physicians India.* 2009;57:345-56.
48. Jackson ML, Nelson JC, Weiss NS, et al. Influenza vaccination and risk of community-acquired pneumonia in immunocompetent elderly people: A population-based, nested case-control study. *Lancet.* 2008;372(9636):398-405.
49. Johnstone J, Marrie TJ, Eurich DT, et al. Effect of pneumococcal vaccination in hospitalized adults with community-acquired pneumonia. *Arch Intern Med.* 2007;167(18):1938-43.
50. Lee TA, Weaver FM, Weiss KB. Impact of pneumococcal vaccination on pneumonia rates in patients with COPD and asthma. *J Gen Intern Med.* 2007;22(1):62-7.
51. Musher DM, Rueda AM, Nahm MH, et al. Initial and subsequent response to pneumococcal polysaccharide and protein-conjugate vaccines administered sequentially to adults who have recovered from pneumococcal pneumonia. *J Infect Dis.* 2008;198(7):1019-27.

World Clin Pulm Crit Care Med. 2019;6(1):88-105.

Hospital-acquired and Ventilator-associated Pneumonia

Vijai Kumar Ratnavelu MD DTCD FCCP FAARC FISDA

Department of Pulmonary Medicine, MediCiti Institute of Medical Sciences
Shamirpet, Hyderabad, Telangana, India

ABSTRACT

Hospital-acquired pneumonia (HAP) is a common nosocomial infection and is prevalent in most of the medical and surgical intensive care units. Nosocomial pneumonia that develops among patients on ventilators is called ventilator-associated pneumonia (VAP). Hospital-acquired pneumonia and VAP significantly increases the cost of care and prolong the hospital stay. Clinical findings of HAP and VAP are often shared with many diseases, such as congestive heart failure, pulmonary emboli, pulmonary hemorrhage, primary or metastatic lung carcinomas, leukemias/ lymphomas, pulmonary drug reactions, and radiation pneumonitis. It is important for the clinicians to know the background in which such clinical presentation occurs and to diagnose it early to prevent mortality.

INTRODUCTION

Infectious Diseases Society of America (IDSA) and American Thoracic Society (ATS)[1] have clarified some of the terms used in the earlier (2005) guidelines. The term hospital-acquired pneumonia (HAP) indicates an episode of pneumonia occurring during hospital stay and is not associated with mechanical ventilation. However, the term ventilator-associated pneumonia (VAP) is an episode of pneumonia, while the patient is intubated and being ventilated. These two terms denote two distinct groups.

Email: drvijaipulmo@yahoo.com

The term health care-associated pneumonia (HCAP), introduced a few years back, which incidentally also caused some confusion among the treating clinicians has been discarded. Extreme caution needs to be exercised while using potent antibiotics.

Each hospital needs to create a database of frequent organisms cultured and their antibiogram. This will help avoid use of double antibiotic for Gram-negative infections, and empiric use of methicillin resistant *Staphylococcus aureus* (MRSA) targeted antibiotics for sensitive staphylococcal infections.

DEFINITIONS

Hospital-acquired pneumonia or nosocomial pneumonia is the pneumonia that occurs 48 hours or more after admission and did not appear to be incubating at the time of admission. Ventilator-associated pneumonia is a type of pneumonia that develops more than 48–72 hours after endotracheal intubation.[1]

EPIDEMIOLOGY

Contrary to the general perception, most cases of HAP, do not occur in the intensive care units (ICUs). However, the highest risk of developing HAP is among patients in the ICUs, being intubated and ventilated. Thus, VAP is widely studied and analyzed. Hospital-acquired pneumonia is the second most frequent nosocomial infection after urinary tract infection, and most frequent acquired infection in the ICU.

In the United States, there has been a gradual decline in the reported incidence of VAP cases, in the medical ICUs (MICUs) over a period of 6 years, beginning 2006. National Healthcare Safety Network (NHSN) reported a decline in the incidence of VAP in MICUs, from 3.1 to 0.9, while in the surgical ICUs, it was less impressive, i.e., 5.2–2.0 per 1,000 ventilator days.[2,3]

However, incidence of VAP has not changed much from 2005 to 2013, in patients aged 65 years and above. A generally accepted incidence of VAP in these populations is between 9.7 and 10.8%.[4] The consequences of developing VAP, especially in countries with poor health care systems, is huge. Ventilator-associated pneumonia can increase hospital stay by 2–3 days and the cost of hospital expenses can increase multiple times, depending upon whether it is a government owned or a private owned hospital.[5] Also, VAP is age related. It is reported to be 5 per 1,000 in people less than 35 years, and 15 per 1,000 in patients greater than 65 years of age.

PATHOGENESIS

The oropharynx (Figure 1) always harbors microorganisms. In a study, throat cultures were positive in 3% of medical students, 30% of hospitalized patients and 60% of ICU patients.[6]

There are the regular "normal" potential bacteria and "abnormal" potential bacteria, which are responsible for primary endogenous infections. The abnormal bacteria are not present at admission, but colonized later, which can cause secondary endogenous infection. In 75% of patients bacteria colonize within 48 hours of hospitalization, and these are the abnormal bacteria introduced directly from outside, and responsible for the exogenous infection (VAP).[7] The entry of these hospital based microorganisms is facilitated by the introduction of the endotracheal tube, which effectively bypasses all the natural defense mechanisms of the upper airway. It appears that sicker the patient, greater the colonization. In addition, the other sources of contamination are the reservoirs of bacteria like the nebulizers, humidifiers, and ventilator tubing. Most contamination happens as a result of nonsterile techniques used during nursing care of the patient, especially during suctioning of the endotracheal (ET) tube secretions.[8] Alterations in gastric pH has been a subject of much debate, as normally the acidic pH of the stomach keeps stomach sterile. Sickness, drugs etc. can make it more alkaline and allow bacteria to thrive.

Louis Pasteur, a French chemist who became the founder of microbiology (1822–1895) had stated that "the seed is nothing and the soil is everything."

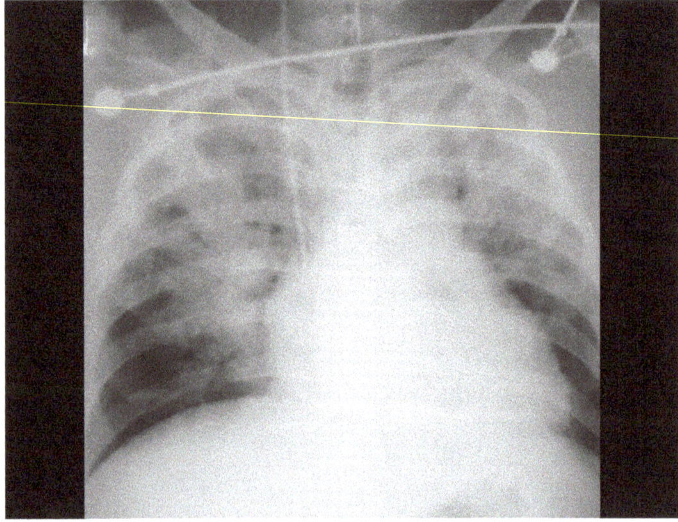

Figure 1: The chest X-ray in a case of ventilator-associated pneumonia.

MICROBIOLOGY

Unlike the community-acquired pneumonia (CAP), where usually a single species of bacteria is responsible for the infection, both HAP and VAP are usually caused by more than one bacterium, sometimes two or even three different bacteria. These polymicrobial pathogens, include aerobic gram-negative bacilli such as *Klebsiella pneumonia*, *Escherichia coli*, *Enterobacter* spp., *Pseudomonas aeruginosa* and *Acinetobacter* spp.; gram-positive cocci such as methicillin sensitive/resistant *Staphylococcus aureus* and *Streptococcus pneumoniae*.[9,10] Are the pathogens different in HAP and VAP? A prospective study[11] conducted in the United States over 3 years in several ICUs, documented 588 episodes in 556 patients: 327 episodes of VAP in 309 patients and 261 episodes of HAP in 247 patients. Among the VAP patients, there were 32% gram-positive cocci, 59% gram-negative bacilli, and 9% miscellaneous pathogens. While in the HAP group, gram-positive cocci were 42.59%, gram-negative bacilli were 39.63% and miscellaneous pathogens were 17.78% (Table 1).

Another study[12] by Kollef et al. evaluated data from 398 ICUs and found similar distribution of pathogens. Although, these studies were done meticulously, it is not wise to extrapolate to different countries with different socioeconomic profiles. It is imperative that every hospital should collect the pattern of ICU pathogens to guide the management strategies.

There were doubts raised about the infections caused by anaerobes in VAP. However, a study which performed anaerobic cultures using protective brush specimens and bronchoalveolar lavage fluid from 185 patients, with a diagnosis of VAP identified just one anaerobic organism, which was a nonpathogenic *Veillonella* spp. This proves that anaerobic cover in the treatment of VAP is unnecessary and a waste of resources.[13]

Table 1: Predominant Organisms Isolated from Hospital-acquired Pneumonia and Ventilator-associated Pneumonia (%)

	Ventilator-associated pneumonia	**Hospital-acquired pneumonia**
Gram-positive	**32**	**42.59**
• Methicillin sensitive *Staphylococcus aureus*	9	13
• Methicillin resistant *Staphylococcus aureus*	18	20
Gram-negative	**59**	**39.63**
• *Pseudomonas*	8	1
• *Stenotrophomonas*	7	9
• *Acinetobacter*	8	13
Miscellaneous	**9**	**17.78**

RISK FACTORS FOR MULTIDRUG-RESISTANT INFECTIONS IN VENTILATOR-ASSOCIATED PNEUMONIA

Risk increases with indiscriminate and empiric use of antibiotics especially in ICUs. Intravenous antibiotics used in the 3 months period before the current hospitalization, patient admitted in a state of shock or acute respiratory distress syndrome (ARDS) prior to the diagnosis of VAP, longer stay (>5 days) in the hospital, and patient having acute kidney injury requiring renal replacement therapy prior to VAP diagnosis are other risk factors.

Chances of developing multidrug resistant (MDR) *Pseudomonas* and other gram-negative bacilli are high in an ICU, where >10% of isolates are resistant to the antibiotic planned. Similarly, for MRSA, possibilities are higher if more than 10% cultures are positive for MRSA.[1] These factors are also the reason for increased mortality.

DIAGNOSIS

The 2016 Clinical Practice Guidelines by the IDSA and the ATS for management of adults with HAP and VAP continues to stress on a clinical diagnosis based on a new radiological infiltrate, which is likely to be of infectious origin such as the new onset of fever, purulent secretions, leukocytosis and hypoxia. When Fàbregas performed autopsy on 25 patients who died while being treated on mechanical ventilator, he found that the above-mentioned features for diagnosis of VAP were good enough, showing a specificity of 75% and sensitivity of 69%.[14]

While a new onset fever, purulent tracheobronchial secretions and hypoxia are easy to be identified early and to raise the suspicion of VAP, a new infiltration on chest X-ray, remains an important proof for the diagnosis of VAP, so much so that a normal X-ray of chest virtually excludes VAP (Figure 1).

There are certain challenges in making a diagnosis of pneumonia, for patient on a ventilator. Factors such as the supine position, anterioposterior view, portable machine, several lines and tubes crisscrossing the chest, and larger heart shadow make the interpretation difficult. In the supine position, the thorax is smaller in volume, as the diaphragm moves cephalad, more so in obese and those receiving neuromuscular blockers. This was proved in a landmark study[15] showing that the position of diaphragm becomes more cephalad in a supine and paralyzed (receiving neuromuscular blockers) patient.

Usual radiological abnormality seen in VAP is alveolar infiltrates. An important feature is the air bronchogram, signifying patent airway with surrounding consolidation. Adjacent solid organs like heart and diaphragm are silhouetted. A parenchymal shadow does not always mean VAP; other pathologies like

ARDS, pleural effusions, noninfective atelectasis, pulmonary thromboembolism, and alveolar hemorrhages are other possibilities. Wundernik et al. autopsied 69 patients who died during mechanical ventilation, and had been diagnosed to have VAP.[16] Out of 69 patients only 24 (35%) had pneumonia on autopsy, and air bronchogram was found to be a reasonably (64%) reliable radiological sign.

SAMPLING LOWER RESPIRATORY TRACT SECRETIONS

Sampling secretions from the lower respiratory tract in a suspected case of VAP is mandatory and essential for making decisions related to antibiotic selection. There are several methods described as follows.

Aspirating Tracheobronchial Secretions

A catheter is introduced into the endotracheal tube as far as it can go, until the resistance is felt, and then suction is applied. The material is collected into a sterile suction trap bottle.

Mini Bronchoalveolar Lavage (Catheter in Catheter Technique)

A large catheter is introduced through the endotracheal tube as far as it can go, then a thinner catheter is threaded through the first catheter, again as far as it can go. This will avoid contamination of the sample. A small amount of saline (5 cc) is flushed into the smaller catheter and then suctioned back into a suction trap bottle. This procedure can easily be done by a trained respiratory therapist or a trained critical care nurse. The test is economical, rapid and can be repeated if required.

Bronchoalveolar Lavage

Bronchoalveolar lavage (BAL) is done by negotiating a flexible bronchoscope into the suspected lobe or segment of the pneumonia as seen on the X-ray of chest. After wedging the tip of the scope, aliquots of 50 mL normal saline are gently pushed into the bronchoscope channel, and aspirated back with manual suctioning. Sequentially, about three aliquots (150 mL) should be sufficient. The suctioned lavage fluid of about 100 mL is considered as a good recovery, which equals sampling of one million alveoli.[17]

Table 2: Thresholds for Different Biological Specimens

Tracheobronchial aspirate	1,000,000 cfu
Bronchoalveolar lavage	10,000 cfu
Protected specimen brushing	1,000 cfu

Protected Specimen Brushing

The protected specimen brushing is introduced through the scope, after it has been wedged into the orifice of the segmental bronchus. At that point, the brush is advanced from inside the sheath, and is brushed against the airway mucosa, thus the brush remains uncontaminated. After brushing, the brush is withdrawn into the sheath and pulled out of the scope.

The sample is subjected to various tests, including Gram stain and pyogenic culture for aerobic bacteria. The presence of large number of neutrophils is consistent with VAP. Kirtland et al. studied the BAL fluid of 39 patients, and concluded that if the fluid had less than 50% neutrophils, BAL had 100% negative predictive value for VAP.[18] Cultures include qualitative, quantitative, and semiquantitative cultures (Table 2).

OTHER TESTS

Procalcitonin (a biological marker) which has been found to be a reliable marker in CAP and sepsis however has no reliable data in relation to VAP. In some studies a steadily rising value of the marker has been found to be associated with septic shock and mortality.[19]

Patients who had a positive culture and have improved with antibiotics, probably have VAP, and the therapy should be continued, but needs to change (or escalate) the antibiotic if the clinical improvement is not as predicted.

On the other hand, patients who had a negative culture are improving, it probably means that they did not have VAP, and antibiotics should be discontinued; however, if these patients are deteriorating, VAP is unlikely and an alternative diagnosis must be found.

DIFFERENTIAL DIAGNOSIS

In the setting where VAP occurs, the diagnosis is made under very difficult circumstances, in a patient with many simultaneous pathologies occurring around the same time. There are many mimics which can confuse the clinician. Pulmonary (chest X-ray) infiltrations, fever and leukocytosis, mucopurulent secretions, and hypoxia can happen in other situations as well. Ventilator-associated pneumonia is commonly misdiagnosed (over diagnosed or under diagnosed) in other clinical situations; they are ARDS, pulmonary thromboembolism, lung contusions, alveolar hemorrhage, lung malignancy, and aspiration pneumonitis due to aspiration of gastric acid. Other rarer disorders are radiation pneumonitis, cryptogenic organizing pneumonia, and drug induced lung disease (e.g., bleomycin induced).

VENTILATOR-ASSOCIATED EVENTS

In view of the inconsistent definitions and variable clinician's perceptions with regards to documentation of the clinical scenarios where VAP is a possibility, Centre for Disease Control (CDC) in 2013 recommended use of the term "ventilator-associated events," which is based on certain occurrences (Table 3). It is too early to judge the usefulness of the new categorization of ventilator-associated complications.

TREATMENT OF VENTILATOR-ASSOCIATED PNEUMONIA

Initially, most VAP require an empiric therapy, and must be started as soon as VAP is suspected, preferably within 1 hour. In order to proceed with empiric antibiotics, it is important to pay attention to the following:

- Every ICU/hospital needs to have their own data of prevailing pathogens and drug susceptibility pattern
- Percentage of gram-negative isolates resistant to an antibiotic being considered
- Each patient's individual risk factors for drug resistance need to be taken into account
- Knowledge of prior antibiotic use. It is better to avoid those which were used recently

Table 3: Ventilator-associated Events

First tier:
- Ventilator-associated condition
- Sustained respiratory deterioration (positive end-expiratory pressure >3 cm H_2O or FiO_2 >0.2 points for 2 days)

Second tier:
- Infection related ventilator-associated complication (IVAC)
- Hyperthermia or hypothermia, leukocytosis or leukopenia, need for starting a new antibiotic

Third tier:
- Possible or probable ventilator-associated pneumonia. Patients who have IVAC also have microbiological evidence of pneumonia

- An initial identification of the pathogen by means of Gram stain of the secretions from respiratory tract
- Antibiotics should cover *Staphylococcus aureus*, *Pseudomonas aeruginosa*, and other gram-negative bacilli.

Treatment of Ventilator-associated Pneumonia with No Known Multidrug Resistance Risk Factors

The following antibiotics are preferred:

- Piperacillin-tazobactam 4.5 g intravenously every 6 hours
- Cefepime 2 g intravenously every 8 hours.

Although, levofloxacin 750 mg intravenously daily was recommended by IDSA/ATS guidelines,[1] many clinicians prefer not to use it in view of its poor action against some gram-negative pathogens.

Treatment of Ventilator-associated Pneumonia with Risk Factors for Multidrug-resistant Pathogen

The patient should receive two antibiotics for *Pseudomonas aeruginosa* and one antibiotic for MRSA. One of the following antibiotics is selected:

- Piperacillin-tazobactam 4.5 g intravenously every 6 hours
- Cefepime 2 g intravenously every 8 hours
- Ceftazidime 2 g intravenously every 8 hours
- Imipenem 500 mg intravenously every 6 hours
- Meropenem 1 g intravenously every 8 hours.

Plus one of the following aminoglycosides:

- Amikacin 15–20 mg/kg intravenously daily
- Gentamicin 5–7 mg/kg intravenously daily
- Tobramycin 5–7 mg/kg intravenously daily.

Usually an aminoglycoside is administered once a day, even with normal renal function. It is preferable to dose aminoglycosides based on the serum levels measured after 6 hours. Aminoglycosides have poor lung penetration, in addition to causing toxicity to kidneys and hearing.

Quinolones

Among the quinolones, especially fluoroquinolones (like ciprofloxacin and levofloxacin) have antipseudomonal activity, in addition to being an ideal drug for

Legionella infection. Ciprofloxacin is given in the dose of 400 mg every 8 hours, and levofloxacin is given as 750 mg intravenously daily.

Alternate Agents

Colistin or polymyxin B can be used for severely resistant *Pseudomonas, Acinetobacter, Enterobacter,* and *Klebsiella*. Nephrotoxicity of polymyxins is significant especially used in conjunction with aminoglycosides.

To cover *Staphylococcus* including methicillin-resistant *Staphylococcus aureus*, the following can be used:

- Linezolid 600 mg intravenously every 12 hours (can be given orally if patient is able to take)
- Vancomycin 15 mg/kg (based on actual body weight) intravenously every 8–12 hours. Nephrotoxicity should be kept in mind.

De-escalation of Antibiotics

As soon as the causative organism is identified by means of a proper culture and sensitivity test, all broad spectrum antibiotics should either be stopped, altered according to the report, and a narrow spectrum antibiotic should be selected.[20] Antibiotics for *Pseudomonas* are an exception. The treatment must be continued with at least two agents. If culture grows nonresistant *Staphylococcus* and nonresistant gram-negative pathogen (from a good sample of secretions), all antibiotics directed toward drug resistant bacteria should be withdrawn. Although, there are no randomized trials, observational studies have not shown any adverse outcomes in the form of increased mortality, or increased duration of ICU stay.[21]

Duration of Antibiotic Therapy

Several studies and meta-analysis has shown that a shorter course of 7 days is as good as a longer duration antibiotic course of 10–15 days.[22,23]

TREATMENT OF HOSPITAL-ACQUIRED PNEUMONIA

Patients who have HAP are less ill compared to patients with VAP. Most patients require only a single antibiotic which can cover *Pseudomonas aeruginosa* and other gram-negative pathogen.[1] Very few might require double antibiotic cover. In order to make this decision, the clinician needs to be familiar with prevailing pathogens in the ICU and hospital, prevailing MDR pathogen frequency, and data of sensitivity to various antibiotics is vital. Most patients of HAP are eminently treatable; however, a small subset of patients have poor prognosis.

Hospital-acquired Pneumonia with Multidrug Resistance Possibility for Gram-negative Bacilli and/or Methicillin-resistant *Staphylococcus aureus*

Such patients should receive two antibiotics directed towards gram-negative bacilli including *Pseudomonas aeruginosa* and one antibiotic directed toward MRSA. It is advisable to select one from each of these two groups:

Group 1

- Piperacillin-tazobactam 4.5 g intravenously every 6 hours
- Cefepime 2 g intravenously every 8 hours
- Ceftazidime 2 g intravenously every 8 hours
- Imipenem 500 mg intravenously every 6 hours
- Meropenem 1 g intravenously every 8 hours.

Although, some guidelines have recommended aztreonam, resistance of gram-negative bacteria to this antibiotic is high.

Group 2

- Amikacin 15–20 mg/kg intravenously daily
- Gentamicin 5–7 mg/kg intravenously daily
- Tobramycin 5–7 mg/kg intravenously daily.

As a rule, aminoglycosides can be dosed once a day even to those with normal renal functions, as these are concentration dependent antibiotics. One single peak in serum concentration is bactericidal.

A few important facts that clinicians need to keep in mind while administering aminoglycosides are:

- Poor lung penetration
- Increased risk of renal toxicity
- Increased risk of ototoxicity
- Not recommended as monotherapy
- After a culture result, withdraw aminoglycoside, if not in the list
- Aminoglycosides can be stopped after 2 or 3 days, if patient improves clinically, and culture shows bacteria that is susceptible to one of the β-lactams.

The IDSA/ATS guidelines recommend either a fluoroquinolone with anti-pseudomonal activity or an aminoglycoside as a second agent for gram-negative bacilli. The guidelines advise to avoid aminoglycosides if alternative agents with good activity against gram-negative bacilli are available. However, many clinicians prefer an aminoglycoside over a fluoroquinolone. The only caveat perhaps is if *Legionella* is a possibility.

For MRSA, one agent may be selected from the following group:

Group 3

- Linezolid 600 mg intravenously every 12 hours (can be given orally if patient is able to take)
- Vancomycin 15 mg/kg every 8–12 hours for patients with normal renal function, with an aim to achieve serum trough concentration of 15–20 μg/mL. A loading dose of 25–30 mg/kg can be given in very sick patients.

Telavancin 10 mg/kg intravenously every 24 hours can be used if the above antibiotics could not be used.[24,25] Food and Drug Administration has given boxed warning for telavancin, that it caused higher mortality in HAP/VAP patients with pre-existing renal impairment. It can cause renal impairment in patients who had normal renal function to begin with; hence, creatinine clearance should be constantly monitored in patients receiving telavancin. Use of telavancin should be avoided in pregnant patients, due to potential risks to fetus.

PROGNOSIS

Analysis of a large number of patients retrospectively by Kollef et al. pointed that mortality rates were 10% in patients with CAP, 19% in patients with HAP, 20% in patients with HCAP, and 29% in patients with VAP.[26] Although, mortality is higher among patients with HAP/VAP, not all of it is due to pneumonia, as these patients have multiple comorbidities and underlying diseases.

All-cause mortality associated with VAP has ranged from 20 to 50% in different studies.[1] In another very large meta-analysis of 24 trials with 6284 patients, the overall attributable mortality was 13%.[27] The mortality was higher among the surgical patients. The mortality was also higher in sicker patients as measured by acute physiology and chronic health evaluation (APACHE) score and simplified acute physiology (SAPS 2) score.

PREVENTION OF HOSPITAL-ACQUIRED PNEUMONIA/VENTILATOR-ASSOCIATED PNEUMONIA

Integrity and effectiveness of any ICU is measured by the risk reduction for nosocomial pneumonia. In order to reduce the risk for HAP/VAP, and the mortality that follows in large number of patients, many important interventions have been recommended, conveniently named as ventilator bundles. Even after many studies demonstrated a reduction in the incidence of HAP/VAP, many clinicians started questioning the value of some of these interventions within these bundles.

It is clear that bacteria enter the lungs from the contaminated hands of the care giver. It may be noted that these hands are contaminated with some of the deadliest bacteria which have learnt to survive the heavy exposure of multiple antibiotics, many of them considered highly bactericidal. Infectious Diseases Society of America and Society of Health Care Epidemiology (SHEA) in 2014 recommended these bundles.[1] Recent reviews are critically looking at the study data and loud thinking if VAP has come down due to these prevention bundles. Metersky et al. analyzed 80,000 charts (2006–2012) as part of audits from Medicare Patient Safety Monitoring System and concluded that VAP has been stable at 10/100 ventilated patients, contrary to CDC reports.[4]

Preventing Aspiration

Since aspiration is a predisposing mechanism for both HAP and VAP, preventing pooling of secretions in the subglottic area around the endotracheal tube and patient positioning are two major activities. It is also important not to damage the tracheal mucosa by causing ischemic necrosis by maintaining the cuff pressure above the capillary filling pressure (around 20–30 cm H_2O) and judicious use of positive end-expiratory pressure.

Avoiding intubation when possible: Use of noninvasive ventilation in respiratory failure due to severe chronic obstructive pulmonary disease is an ideal example.

Subglottic Drainage of Secretions

A meta-analysis of 2,442 patients in 13 randomized trials showed that subglottic secretion drainage reduces VAP;[28] however, of 13 trials some used intermittent suction and some used continuous suction, the outcomes were similar. A recent review by Klompas[29] who was part of 2014 guidelines questions the validity of these studies and concludes "On balance then, the benefits of subglottic secretion drainage appear to be more modest than previously suspected."

Position of patient—It is assumed that making the patient lying flat on bed, increases chances of aspiration, while raising the head side of the bed by 30–45° will minimize the chances of aspiration.

Patient Positioning

Supine positioning appears to predispose to micro-aspiration of the gastric contents and the development of HAP. The head of the bed should therefore be elevated to 30–45°.[4] The evidence was so strong that a trial of 90 intubated patients had to be stopped midway as it became clear that elevation of head side of the patient, did indeed reduce VAP.[30,31] However, many started questioning the outcomes of the studies and as a result a Spanish group tried lateral Trendelenburg position.

The VAP was less, but there were no differences between groups in duration of mechanical ventilation, ICU length-of-stay, or hospital mortality.

Decontamination of the Digestive Tract

It is assumed that the esophagus and nasopharynx are colonized with organisms, sometimes MDR organisms. These organisms can travel and colonize in the respiratory tract. Decontamination of the digestive tract can reduce the incidence of pneumonia in intubated patients by decreasing colonization of the upper respiratory tract. This can be achieved by washing the oropharynx with antiseptics like chlorhexidine and selective decontamination of the oropharynx with nonabsorbable antibiotics.

Poor oral hygiene has been an issue in the elderly, more so when they are intubated. Chlorhexidine 0.12% oral solution (15 mL twice daily until 24 hours after extubation) is a good recommendation. Using antibiotics for this purpose has not found favor at many centers. Incidence of VAP with proper oral care, has been brought down as shown by a meta-analysis done in the year 2007, which included 3242 patients gathered from 11 trials and showed a risk reduction (RR) of 0.56, 95% CI.[32]

Gastric Ulcer Prevention and Avoiding Antacids/Proton Pump Inhibitors

The pH of gastric juice is always acidic. When the pH changes to less acidic, there is a greater chance of colonization and VAP. Studies compared ranitidine, aluminum hydroxide/magnesium hydroxide, and sucralfate; and found that sucralfate results in lesser number of VAP (5 with sucralfate and 21 with ranitidine).[33]

Probiotics

Probiotics did not result in any reduction in the incidence of VAP, use of antibiotics, duration of mechanical ventilation, length of hospital stay, or mortality.

Spontaneous Awakening and Spontaneous Breathing Trials

Spontaneous awakening trials (SAT) and spontaneous breathing trials (SBT) were both associated with significantly less time to extubation and lower ventilator-mortality rates.[34] Spontaneous breathing trials were also associated with lower hazards for ventilator-associated events, including infection related ventilator-associated complications. These findings confirm the findings of randomized controlled trials demonstrating that SAT and SBT can decrease mean duration of mechanical ventilation, ICU length of stay, and even mortality, particularly when these two maneuvers are combined together.[35-38]

Glucocorticoids

Some studies[39] have shown beneficial effects and some other studies[40] have not shown any benefit in preventing HAP/VAP in critically ill patients. More studies are needed to define the role of steroids. There has been no mortality benefit in either scenario. Hydrocortisone 200 mg intravenously once a day for 5 days, followed by 100 mg on 6th day and then 50 mg on the 7th day was used.

Oral Care with Chlorhexidine

Regular chlorhexidine mouth wash has been a part of VAP bundle. However, recent evidence points to increased mortality, although VAP incidence is less.[41,42] The reasons are not clear. It is speculated that it could be an ARDS caused by trickling of chlorhexidine into the lungs. Perhaps it may be best to provide oral care without chlorhexidine.[43]

Other Measures

- Hand washing of all staff and caregivers involved in providing care to patients on ventilator (before and after touching any part of the patient, the ventilator or the endotracheal tube)
- Minimizing transport while ventilated (when feasible)
- Implementation of weaning protocols
- Minimizing sedation
- Maintaining and improving physical conditioning
- Maintaining ventilator circuits
- Early liberation from mechanical ventilator.

CONCLUSION

The care of patient on a mechanical ventilator is a continuum, which starts with intubation and ends with extubation. The mindset and work culture of caregivers around the patient is important. The quality of care needs to be provided in all shifts and on all days, aiming to liberate the patient at the earliest. This needs to be achieved without much sedation and focusing on SAT and SBT.

Editor's Comment

Hospital-acquired pneumonia (HAP) and ventilator-associated pneumonia (VAP) are serious illnesses that are seen in most hospitals and are associated with high mortality. This will increase the hospital stay of the patient and contribute to increased mortality. The profile of organisms causing HAP and VAP is very different from those causing community-acquired pneumonia. These infections are often polymicrobial and mostly caused by drug resistant organisms. Early identification of pathogen causing HAP and VAP is very important to guide appropriate antibiotic therapy. The clinical pulmonary infection score has been widely used for the diagnosis of nosocomial pneumonia. Once diagnosed, these infections require early and aggressive antibiotic therapy. Choice of antibiotic should be guided by antimicrobial data of the ICU or ward. If possible monotherapy with appropriate antibiotic should be initiated. If multiple higher antibiotics are started early, de-escalation is to be tried to avoid emergence of antibiotic resistance and to reduce cost of therapy. Every ICU should develop protocols for infection control and this is to be strictly implemented.

Ravindran Chetambath

REFERENCES

1. Kalil AC, Metersky ML, Klompas M et al. Management of adults with hospital-acquired and ventilator-associated pneumonia: 2016 clinical practice guidelines by the Infectious Diseases Society of America and the American Thoracic Society. *Clin Infect Dis.* 2016;63(5):e61-111.
2. Edwards JR, Peterson KD, Andrus ML, et al. National Healthcare Safety Network (NHSN) Report, data summary for 2006, issued June 2007. *Am J Infect Control.* 2007;35:290-331.
3. Dudeck MA, Weiner LM, Allen-Bridson K, et al. National Healthcare Safety Network (NHSN) report, data summary for 2012, device-associated module. *Am J Infect Control.* 2013;41:1148-66.
4. Metersky ML, Wang Y, Klompas M, et al. Trend in ventilator-associated pneumonia rates between 2005 and 2013. *JAMA.* 2016;316:2427-29.
5. Kollef MH, Hamilton CW, Ernst FR. Economic impact of ventilator-associated pneumonia in a large matched cohort. *Infect Control Hosp Epidemiol.* 2012;33:250-6.
6. Johanson WG, Pierce AK, Sanford JP. Changing pharyngeal bacterial flora of hospitalized patients. Emergence of gram-negative bacilli. *N Engl J Med.* 1969;281(21):1137-40.
7. Garrouste-Orgeas M, Chevret S, Arlet G, et al. Oropharyngeal or gastric colonization and nosocomial pneumonia in adult intensive care unit patients. A prospective study based on genomic DNA analysis. *Am J Respir Crit Care Med.* 1997;156:1647-55.
8. Nseir S, Di Pompeo C, Pronnier P, et al. Nosocomial tracheobronchitis in mechanically ventilated patients: incidence, aetiology and outcome. *Eur Respir J.* 2002;20:1483-9.
9. Jones RN. Microbial etiologies of hospital-acquired bacterial pneumonia and ventilator-associated bacterial pneumonia. *Clin Infect Dis.* 2010;51(Suppl. 1):S81-7.

10. Sievert DM, Ricks P, Edwards JR, et al. Antimicrobial-resistant pathogens associated with healthcare-associated infections: summary of data reported to the National Healthcare Safety Network at the Centers for Disease Control and Prevention, 2009-2010. *Infect Control Hosp Epidemiol.* 2013;34:1-14.
11. Weber DJ, Rutala WA, Sickbert-Bennett EE, et al. Microbiology of ventilator-associated pneumonia compared with that of hospital-acquired pneumonia. *Infect Control Hosp Epidemiol.* 2007;28:825-31.
12. Kollef MH, Morrow LE, Niederman MS, et al. Clinical characteristics and treatment patterns among patients with ventilator-associated pneumonia. *Chest.* 2006;129(5):1210-18.
13. Marik PE, Careau P. The role of anaerobes in patients with ventilator-associated pneumonia and aspiration pneumonia: a prospective study. *Chest.* 1999;115:178-83.
14. Fàbregas N, Ewig S, Torres A, et al. Clinical diagnosis of ventilator associated pneumonia revisited: comparative validation using immediate post-mortem lung biopsies. *Thorax.* 1999;54(10):867-73.
15. Froese AB, Bryan AC. Effects of anesthesia and paralysis on diaphragmatic mechanics in man. *Anesthesiology.* 1974;41(3):242-55.
16. Wunderink RG, Woldenberg LS, Zeiss J, et al. The radiologic diagnosis of autopsy-proven ventilator-associated pneumonia. *Chest.* 1992;101(2):458-63.
17. Seijo LM, Flandes J, Somiedo MV, et al. A prospective randomized study comparing manual and wall suction in the performance of bronchoalveolar lavage. *Respiration.* 2016;91(6):480-5.
18. Kirtland SH, Corley DE, Winterbauer RH, et al. The diagnosis of ventilator-associated pneumonia: a comparison of histologic, microbiologic, and clinical criteria. *Chest.* 1997;112(2):445-57.
19. Hillas G, Vassilakopoulos T, Plantza P, et al. C-reactive protein and procalcitonin as predictors of survival and septic shock in ventilator-associated pneumonia. *Eur Respir J.* 2010;35(4):805-11.
20. Ewig S. Nosocomial pneumonia: De-escalation is what matters. *Lancet Infect Dis.* 2011;11:155-7.
21. Leone M, Bechis C, Baumstarck K, et al. De-escalation versus continuation of empirical antimicrobial treatment in severe sepsis: a multicenter non-blinded randomized noninferiority trial. *Intensive Care Med.* 2014;40:1399-408.
22. Pugh R, Grant C, Cooke RP, et al. Short-course versus prolonged-course antibiotic therapy for hospital-acquired pneumonia in critically ill adults. *Cochrane Database Syst Rev.* 2015;8:CD007577.
23. Chastre J, Wolff M, Fagon JY, et al. Comparison of 8 vs 15 days of antibiotic therapy for ventilator-associated pneumonia in adults: a randomized trial. *JAMA.* 2003;290:2588-98.
24. VIBATIV (Telavancin) - Highlights of prescribing information. Available from: https://www.vibativ.com/public/pdf/PrescribingInformation.pdf
25. Rubinstein E, Lalani T, Corey GR, et al. (ATTAIN Study Group) Telavancin versus vancomycin for hospital-acquired pneumonia due to Gram-positive pathogens. *Clin Infect Dis.* 2011;52(1):31-40.
26. Kollef MH, Shorr A, Tabak YP, et al. Epidemiology and outcomes of health-care-associated pneumonia: results from a large US database of culture-positive pneumonia. *Chest.* 2005;128(6):3784-7.
27. Melsen WG, Rovers MM, Groenwold RH, et al. Attributable mortality of ventilator-associated pneumonia: A meta-analysis of individual patient data from randomised prevention studies. *Lancet Infect Dis.* 2013; 13(8):665-71.
28. Muscedere J, Rewa O, McKechnie K, et al. Subglottic secretion drainage for the prevention of ventilator-associated pneumonia: a systematic review and meta-analysis. *Crit Care Med.* 2011;39:1985-91.
29. Klompas M, Branson R, Eichenwald EC, et al. Strategies to prevent ventilator-associated pneumonia in acute care hospitals: 2014 update. *Infect Control Hosp Epidemiol.* 2014;35(8):915-36.
30. Klompas M. What is new in the prevention of nosocomial pneumonia in the ICU? *Curr Opin Crit Care.* 2017;23(5):378-84.
31. Torres A, Serra-Batlles J, Ros E, et al. Pulmonary aspiration of gastric contents in patients receiving mechanical ventilation: The effect of body position. *Ann Intern Med.* 1992;116(7):540-3.
32. Orozco-Levi M, Torres A, Ferrer M, et al. Semirecumbent position protects from pulmonary aspiration but not completely from gastroesophageal reflux in mechanically ventilated patients. *Am J Respir Crit Care Med.* 1995;152:1387-90.

33. Chan EY, Ruest A, Meade MO, et al. Oral decontamination for prevention of pneumonia in mechanically ventilated adults: Systematic review and meta-analysis. *BMJ.* 2007;334(7599):889.
34. Prod'hom G, Leuenberger P, Koerfer J, et al. Nosocomial pneumonia in mechanically ventilated patients receiving antacid, ranitidine, or sucralfate as prophylaxis for stress ulcer. A randomized controlled trial. *Ann Intern Med.* 1994;120(8):653-62.
35. Klompas M, Li L, Kleinman K, et al. Associations between ventilator bundle components outcomes. *JAMA Intern Med.* 2016;176:1277-83.
36. Esteban A, Frutos F, Tobin MJ, et al. A comparison of four methods of weaning patients from mechanical ventilation. Spanish Lung Failure Collaborative Group. *N Engl J Med.* 1995;332:345-50.
37. Ely EW, Baker AM, Dunagan DP, et al. Effect on the duration of mechanical ventilation of identifying patients capable of breathing spontaneously. *N Engl J Med.* 1996;335:1864-9.
38. Kress JP, Pohlman AS, O'Connor MF, Hall JB. Daily interruption of sedative infusions in critically ill patients undergoing mechanical ventilation. *N Engl J Med.* 2000;342:1471-7.
39. Girard TD, Kress JP, Fuchs BD, et al. Efficacy and safety of a paired sedation and ventilator weaning protocol for mechanically ventilated patients in intensive care (awakening and breathing controlled trial): A randomised controlled trial. Lancet. 2008;371:126-34.
40. Roquilly A, Mahe PJ, Seguin P, et al. Hydrocortisone therapy for patients with multiple traumas: The randomized controlled HYPOLYTE study. *JAMA.* 2011;305(12):1201-9.
41. Bulger EM, Cuschieri J. Steroids after severe injury: many unanswered questions. *JAMA.* 2011;305:1242-3.
42. Klompas M, Speck K, Howell MD, et al. Reappraisal of routine oral care with chlorhexidine gluconate for patients receiving mechanical ventilation: Systematic review and meta-analysis. *JAMA Internal Med.* 2014;174:751-61.
43. Price R, MacLennan G, Glen J. Selective digestive or oropharyngeal decontamination and topical oropharyngeal chlorhexidine for prevention of death in general intensive care: Systematic review and network meta-analysis. *BMJ.* 2014;348:g2197.

World Clin Pulm Crit Care Med. 2019;6(1):106-20.

Pneumonia in Immunocompromised Host

George D'Souza MD DNB

Department of Pulmonary Medicine, St John's Medical College
Bengaluru, Karnataka, India

ABSTRACT

An immunocompromised host (ICH) is vulnerable to infections and the lung is an important organ involved. Seventy percent of lung infiltrates are due to infection in an ICH and an important cause for morbidity and mortality. The type of immune defect predisposes to specific infections some of which are opportunistic. Understanding the type of immunosuppression and the setting in which pneumonia develops is important to predict the etiology and make an early diagnosis. Radiology is important in identifying infection but does not help in identifying the causative agents. Bronchoscopy and transthoracic aspiration are useful in establishing the diagnosis. Prophylaxis and vaccines may help reduce infections in the immunocompromised.

INTRODUCTION

An immunocompromised host is defined as one who has an increased risk for life-threatening infection because of a congenital or acquired defect in immune status.[1] The lung is vulnerable to infection because of its constant and continuous contact with the environment. In a normal adult, around 600 L of air moves in and out in an hour, and this is brought into contact with a surface size of a tennis court. In immunocompetent individuals, the body's immune system—innate and acquired, does well to protect the lungs. When these are lacking or break down, the lung becomes vulnerable to infection. Today, there is widespread use

Email: Dsouza.ga1975@gmail.com

of immunosuppression for a variety of conditions like autoimmune disorders, collagen vascular disorders, transplant etc. In addition, chemotherapy used in malignancy with its effects on white blood cells also predisposes to lung infection.[2] Infections are responsible for over three fourths of the pulmonary complications in the immunocompromised.[3]

Diabetes mellitus, a common condition, also needs to be remembered as a cause for immunosuppression, particularly when uncontrolled.[4] Along with the increasing prevalence of diabetes, this becomes probably the largest population of immunocompromised subjects. It is now well accepted that it increases the risk of pneumonia and tuberculosis (TB).[5,6] Fungal infections are also not rare.[7]

An immunocompromised patient is susceptible to not only infections with virulent organisms but also less virulent organisms to which a person with normal immunity is unlikely to be susceptible. The local tissue response is also muted and hence, both the clinical and radiological presentations will be different from those with intact immunity. A classic example is the presentation of TB in those with normal immunity and those with acquired immunodeficiency syndrome. The vulnerability to infections and the type of infection is also dependent upon the type and the severity of immune deficiency.

Early diagnosis and treatment is critical to decrease morbidity and mortality in this vulnerable group of patients.[8] Understanding the relationship between the type, and severity of immunodeficiency and the susceptibility to specific pathogens with their clinical and radiological presentation is important to diagnose and treat these patients.[9]

HOST DEFENSES—INNATE AND ACQUIRED

To tackle the lungs vulnerability to infection, the lung has a primitive system which is broad based called the innate immune system, and a more sophisticated and refined system called the adaptive immune system. The innate system has evolved to recognize certain molecular patterns on microbes called "pathogen associated molecular patterns," which includes carbohydrates, lipids, and deoxyribonucleic acid/ribonucleic acid sequences. The system has evolved to recognize harmless substances while retaining the capacity to mount a robust response to harmful substances particularly pathogenic microbes. It is also critical in priming the acquired system. The system involves the epithelium of the airways and alveoli; dendritic cells and their precursors; and recruited neutrophils and monocytes. These work in a coordinated fashion and form the first defense of the lung, tolerating harmless inhaled substances and self-antigens and mounting a response to pathogens and noxious substances. They are also integral to the final resolution of injury and restoration of lung function.[10]

The adaptive immune response is primarily provided by the lymphocytes; B-cells which are derived from the bone marrow, T-cells from the thymus, and natural killer (NK) cells. The T-cells have "T-cell receptors" which differentiate them. The B-cells have "surface immunoglobulin" which differentiate them, while the NK cells has none. Activation of T-cells is critical to the acquired immune response. The T-cell population can be broadly divided into helper and suppressor. The helper T-cells are divided into Th1, Th2, and Th17 according to their secreted cytokine profile and have specific functions; Th1 is responsible for cell mediated immune response, Th2 interact with B-cells to help switch class to produce immunoglobulin G (IgG) antibodies and Th17 act as the interface between the innate and adaptive immune systems. The B-cells are responsible for the humoral response.[11]

For practical purposes the defects in the immune system can be grouped into five broad categories: (i) defect in phagocytes, (ii) humoral defects, (iii) defects in cell mediated immunity, (iv) defects in complement, and (v) defects secondary to splenectomy or hyposplenism (Table 1).[12] Sometimes, a patient may have more than one defect.

Table 1: Potential Infections According to Immune Defect

Immune defect or deficiency	Bacteria	Fungus	Virus	Parasite
Phagocytic	*S. aureus, E. coli, P. aeruginosa, K. pneumoniae*	*Aspergillus* and *Candida*		
B-cell defects	*S. pneumoniae, H. influenzae, P. aeruginosa*			
T-cell defects	Mycobacteria, *Nocardia, Legionella*	*Cryptococcus neoformans, Histoplasma capsulatum, Coccidioides immitis, P. jirovecii*	CMV, Varicella, HSV	*T. gondii*
Splenectomy/ hyposplenism	Capsulated organisms like *S. pneumoniae, S. aureus, H. influenzae*	*Aspergillus* species, *Candida* species, *Histoplasma capsulatum*		
Corticosteroids	*S. aureus, Legionella, P. aeruginosa* and other gram-negative bacteria, mycobacteria, *Nocardia*		CMV, Varicella, HSVP	

CMV, cytomegalovirus; HSV, herpes simplex virus, HSVP, herpes simplex virus pneumonia.

Dysfunction of Phagocytes

It could be quantitative or qualitative. Neutropenia is probably the most important cause. It is seen in patients with leukemia, marrow failure, and because of chemotherapy. There are also important but relatively rare qualitative conditions like chronic granulomatous disease and Job's syndrome. In the former, the granulocyte is unable to kill catalase positive organisms resulting in severe recurrent infections. It usually presents in the first year of life. In Job's syndrome characterized by increase in IgE and eosinophilia, neutrophil migration is affected. Patients are susceptible to *Staphylococcus*, gram-negative aerobic organisms, and fungal infections particularly *Aspergillus* and *Candida*. Infection with *Nocardia asteroides* is also not uncommon.

B-cell Defects

These are responsible for the humoral or antibody response to infection. They protect by either neutralizing the organisms or by opsonization, which facilitates phagocytosis and killing through activation of complement. Defects or deficiency predisposes the individual to infection with capsulated organisms like pneumococcus, *H. influenzae*, meningococcus, and *P. aeruginosa*. Antibody deficiency may be primary or secondary. Primary antibody deficiency is seen in common variable immunodeficiency, X-linked agammaglobulinemia, and selective IgA or IgM deficiency. Secondary causes are seen in multiple myeloma, Waldenstrom macroglobulinemia, and chronic lymphocytic leukemia. They predispose to recurrent pneumonias which may ultimately lead to bronchiectasis.[13,14]

T-cells Defects

These are important for both cell mediated and humoral immune responses. Reduction in CD4 lymphocytes can affect Th1 responses and Th2 responses. The former predisposes to infections which need macrophage activation like TB, *Pneumocystis jirovecii* etc., and the latter predisposes to infections that need the humoral response. CD8 lymphocytes are important in eliminating host cells infected with pathogens typically seen in viral infections.[15] Defects in T-cell function can thus predispose to a wide spectrum of infection including bacteria, fungi, viruses, and parasites as seen in those who are infected by human immunodeficiency virus (HIV). They are particularly susceptible to intracellular pathogens like *Legionella* spp., *Nocardia, Cryptococcus neoformans, Histoplasma capsulatum*, herpes simplex, cytomegalovirus (CMV), Epstein–Barr virus (EBV), *Pneumocystis jirovecii*, and *Toxoplasma gondii*. Human immunodeficiency virus is the most common cause of acquired T-cell immunodeficiency. Others are drug induced, malnutrition, lymphoma, and hairy cell leukemia. Primary causes are less common and are usually hereditary like Wiskott-Aldrich syndrome, ataxia-telangiectasia, DiGeorge syndrome, etc. Patients are predisposed to frequent opportunistic infections including *Mycobacterium tuberculosis* and nontuberculous mycobacteria, CMV, *Pneumocystis jirovecii*, etc.

Defects in the Complement System

Complement activation is a step in the opsonization of bacteria which facilitates phagocytosis and killing of extracellular bacteria. Complement defects are usually primary and include deficiencies of C3, C5, C6, C7, C8, and C9, which predisposes to recurrent infections with encapsulated organisms like *Pneumococcus*, *N. gonorrhoeae*, and *N. meningitides*.[16]

Splenic Dysfunction

Spleen is the largest lymphoid tissue in the body. It produces opsonizing antibodies and removes antibody coated organisms from the bloodstream. Patients who have undergone splenectomy or who have splenic dysfunction, as seen in Hodgkin's disease are susceptible to overwhelming infection with capsulated organisms like *S. pneumoniae, H. influenzae*, and *S. aureus*.[17]

RADIOLOGY IN THE DIAGNOSIS OF IMMUNOCOMPROMISED PNEUMONIA

Chest X-ray

It is usually the first step in the identification and diagnosis of lung infection (Figure 1A). The findings usually are not specific to give a definitive etiological diagnosis. However, the "clinical setting" comprising the epidemiological setting, the type, severity, and duration of immune deficit along with the radiological pattern may help in narrowing the probable etiological agent.[2]

In countries like India where TB prevalence is high, TB would be an important differential diagnosis. Similarly, in areas where the endemic fungi are prevalent, fungal disease would be an important differential diagnosis. A history of recent travel to an area endemic for an infection along with a typical radiological picture could help clinch the diagnosis or suggest a diagnostic test.

The duration of immunosuppression is also helpful to narrow the potential causative organisms (Table 2). In a neutropenic, for example, infections in the first week are caused by usual pathogens like gram-negative bacteria or *S. aureus*. After the second week, fungal infections like Aspergillus become important.[18] In

Table 2: Potential Pathogens According to Duration of Immunosuppression

Clinical conditions	Early (<1 month)	Intermediate (1–6 months)	Late (>6 months)
Neutropenia	Bacterial—community and hospital-acquired	Fungal	–
Solid organ transplant	Hospital-acquired—bacterial, HSV, *Candida*	Fungal; viral—CMV RSV, HSV, adenovirus, and influenza; *M. tuberculosis; Nocardia*	Community-acquired pneumonia, viral-influenza, adenovirus, RSV, endemic fungi, *H. capsulatum*
Stem cell transplant	*Aspergillus*	CMV, PJP, *Aspergillus*	Bacteria, fungal, viral—RSV, VZV, parainfluenza

CMV, Cytomegalovirus; HSV, Herpes simplex virus; PJP, *Pneumocystis jirovecii* pneumonia; RSV, respiratory syncytial virus; VZV, varicella zoster virus.

those undergoing solid organ transplant, three periods can be identified; the first month when most infections are due to those seen in normal patients undergoing surgery and are due to oral flora, gram-negative bacilli, and secondary to emboli from infected lines. In the next 1–6 months, viruses dominate. Viruses also worsen immunosuppression and predispose to *P. jirovicii* and fungal infections. After 6 months, the status of the graft determines the type of infection.[19] Those who have good function have infections like that of nonimmunocompromised hosts, while in those who have poor graft function requiring high doses of immunosuppression, opportunistic infections are common. A small number (5–10%) develop chronic viral infections, particularly EBV which results in organ failure or lymphoproliferative malignancies or both.[20,21] Tuberculosis secondary to reactivation is an important infection during this period and seen in 0.5–2% of patients. In endemic areas like India, it may be as high as 15% of transplant patients.[22]

Broadly, radiological shadows due to infections cause four patterns or a combination of the same—consolidation, bronchopneumonia, nodules, and diffuse lung disease.[2,23] These patterns are useful but not diagnostic and help narrow the possibilities (Table 3). Consolidation is usually seen in bacterial infections and occasionally in mycobacterial. It may be lobar, segmental, or subsegmental in its distribution. Occasionally, it can involve a whole hemithorax. Atypical organisms like *Legionella*, *Mycoplasma*, etc. can also cause consolidation but are more likely to present with patchy opacifications which is multifocal and bilateral.[24] The rate of progression may help to narrow the possible causative organisms; an acute presentation is more likely to be a bacterial infection while

Table 3: Pathogen According to Radiological Presentation and Progression

Pattern	Acute	Subacute/chronic
Consolidation	Bacterial	Mycobacteria, fungi
Nodule(s)	Septic emboli, *Legionella*	Mycobacteria, *Nocardia*, fungal infection
Diffuse	*Mycobacterium tuberculosis*, disseminated fungal infection	Viruses, *P. jirovicii*

a subacute or chronic progression is seen in fungal, *P. jirovicii*, mycobacterial, nocardial and viral infections like CMV.[19] Bronchopneumonia is usually due to aspiration from colonized upper airways and causes patchy opacities which are multifocal and centered in distal airways. The organisms are usually *S. aureus*, *Pseudomonas aeruginosa*, and gram-negative organisms which colonize the upper airways.[24] Nodules which may be single or multiple with or without cavitation are seen in tuberculosis, nocardiosis, and fungal infections.[25] It is also seen in septic emboli and *Legionella*. An air crescent sign or a hallo sign may be seen and is suggestive of aspergillosis. It is due to the angio-invasive nature of the infection causing infarction and necrosis in the center with a surrounding area of hemorrhage.[26] Diffuse or interstitial pattern are seen in viral infections and *P. jirovicii*. In *P. jirovicii* infection, there may also be interstitial thickening giving the classical crazy pavement like pattern.

Computed Tomography Thorax

It may be more useful in narrowing the diagnosis as it provides more details. It is particularly useful in diagnosing fungal infections and *P. jirovicii* infections. It is not so useful in differentiating the causes of consolidation.[27] Diffuse ground glass opacities with centrilobular nodule with or without patchy areas of consolidation is seen in CMV infection,[28] while HSV is characterized by multifocal ground glass opacities or peribronchial consolidation or both.[29] *P. jirovecii* infection is characterized by diffuse ground glass with occasional nodules or cysts and interstitial thickening. Computed tomography (CT) is superior to conventional X-rays in demonstrating cavitation as seen in fungal infections and TB.[23] In fungal infections, cavitation or the presence of air crescent sign are seen and may be missed on a chest X-ray but seen or better visualized on a CT thorax (Figure 1B). This may also be true in pneumonia due to *Staphylococcus aureus*.

The CT is more sensitive in picking up pneumonia particularly in the intensive care unit and in the immunocompromised. Its utility in establishing the diagnosis is only in mycoplasma infection and *P. jirovecii*. In fungal infections, if typical findings are seen, it may help narrow the differential diagnosis. It is also useful to

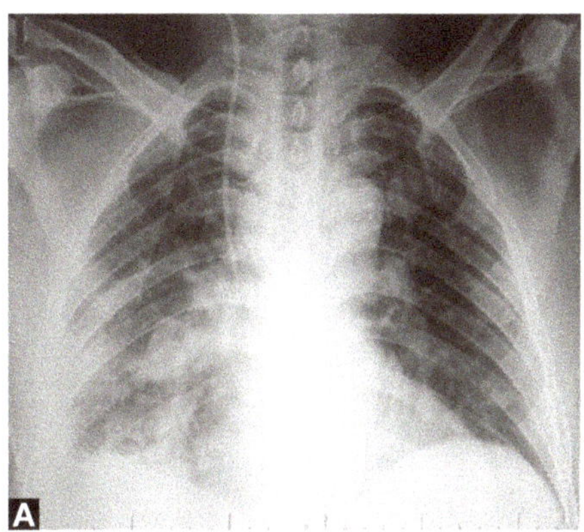

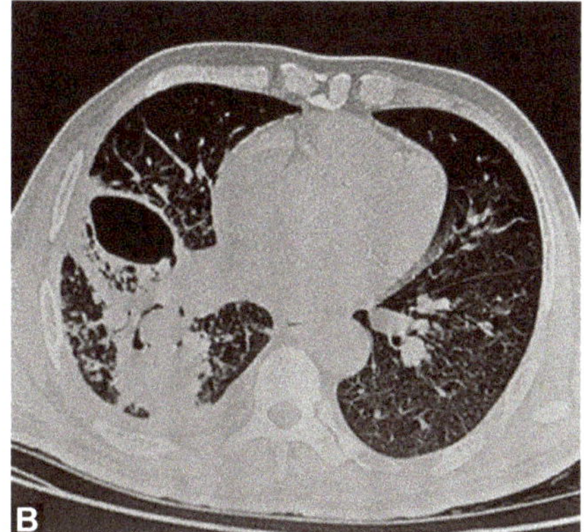

Figure 1: A case of mucormycosis in an uncontrolled diabetic patient. The chest X-ray shows, **A,** right lower zone consolidation, and **B,** computed tomograpgy thorax shows cavities and an air crescent sign.

plan diagnostic procedures like lavage, transbronchial lung biopsy (TBLB), and fine needle aspiration cytology (FNAC) as it helps in better.[23]

It is worth remembering here that although over 70% of shadows in this population of patients are due to infections, they need to be distinguished from noninfectious causes which include pulmonary edema, pulmonary hemorrhage, drug toxicity, and even malignancy.[30] They are most often diffuse and it is critical to differentiate them from infection by appropriate investigations.

Bronchoscopy in the Diagnosis

Using fiber optic bronchoscopy (FOB), one can inspect the airways and take brushings, do a lavage and take TBLB from the affected regions.[31] Bronchial washings, the aspiration of secretions after instillation of saline in the major airway is useful in diagnosing TB and endemic fungal infections particularly when lavage returns are poor. Bronchoalveolar lavage (BAL) is done by instillation of saline aliquots after the bronchoscope is wedged in the area of involvement. It had an overall diagnostic yield of 66% in one study and was particularly useful in infections due to *P. jirovicii*, CMV, fungus, and TB. A protected BAL culture is useful in neutropenic patients not responding to empirical treatment. It is safe even in the presence of thrombocytopenia.[32] Bronchial brushings are useful in viral infections. The cells will show characteristic cytopathic changes and viral inclusion bodies. Transbronchial lung biopsy is useful in *Pneumocystis jirovecii pneumonia* (PJP), TB, and viral infections. It may help confirm fungal infections by demonstrating tissue invasion. However, the incremental yield is only around 15%.[31] Fiber optic bronchoscopy is the procedure of choice for evaluation of

Table 4: Potential Pathogens According to CD4 Count in Patients Infected with Human Immunodeficiency Virus	
CD4 count	**Potential pathogen**
<100 cell/mm^3	CMV, NTM, histoplasmosis, endemic fungi, toxoplasmosis
<200 cell/mm^3	PJP, disseminated TB
<200 cell/mm^3	Bacterial pneumonia, nocardia, and TB (primary pattern)

CMV, Cytomegalovirus; NTM, Nontuberculous mycobacteria; PJP, *Pneumocystis jirovecii* pneumonia; TB, tuberculosis.

patients with HIV and post solid organ transplant with pulmonary infiltrates. Bronchoalveolar lavage should always be done and TBLB to be done if an incremental yield is expected. If BAL and other procedures including noninvasive tests do not yield a diagnosis, TBLB may be done before subjecting patient to an open lung biopsy. In neutropenic patients, FOB is indicated when there is no response to empirical treatment.[31,33]

SPECIFIC CONDITIONS

Human Immunodeficiency Virus Induced Immunosuppression

It is associated with opportunistic infections which are related to the degree of immunosuppression as reflected by the CD4 count (Table 4). Seventy percent of patients will have a lung infection during the course of their disease. *Pneumocystis jirovecii* pneumonia is the most common infection worldwide.[34] Tuberculosis is the most common infection in India during all stages of the disease although the presentation differs depending on the degree of immunosuppression. The presentation is more like primary or disseminated TB when the CD4 count is low and more like in immunocompetent patients when the CD4 count is high. Extrapulmonary TB is seen in nearly half the patients.[35,36] Prophylaxis, demography, and degree of immunosuppression determine the type of infection. Successful treatment with antiretroviral therapy considerably reduces the risk of developing opportunistic infections.

Patients Receiving Biologicals

These are used in the treatment of autoimmune diseases and hematological malignancies. Rituximab targets B cells while alemtuzumab targets both T- and B-cells. They predispose to an increased risk of developing pneumonias. Alemtuzumab has been associated with PJP, Aspergillus and viral pneumonias. *Pneumocystis jirovecii* pneumonia prophylaxis should be considered.

Anti-tumor necrosis factor-α inhibitors are used in treating patients with rheumatoid arthritis. While they do not increase the risk of pneumonias, they increase the risk for developing granulomatous and intracellular infections like TB, *H. capsulatum, L. pneumophila*, etc. Tuberculosis is often disseminated and usually presents in the first 90 days of treatment. The risk is greater with infliximab than with etanercept. Hence, it is advisable to screen for latent TB in those who are being initiated on treatment with one of these agents.[37,38]

Long-term Oral Glucocorticoid

It is defined as a dose greater than 5–10 mg/day taken by 1.2% and 0.75% of the adult population in United States and United Kingdom, respectively. It is likely to be significant in India too. It is associated with an increased risk of developing bacterial infections particularly lower respiratory tract infection and reactivation of TB. A dose greater than 10 mg/day or a cumulative dose greater than 700 mg was associated with a risk over 5 times that of those not on steroids. Steroids may also mask the presentation of infection with systemic symptoms like fever being not so prominent. Hence, patients on long-term oral glucocorticoids need to be closely monitored for infection and attention should be paid to vaccination against pneumonia and flu.[39-41]

Diabetes Mellitus

Diabetes mellitus increases risk of developing infections. The exact mechanism of dysfunction in the immune system is not clear. Animal models have shown dysfunction in neutrophil function while more recent studies have shown decreased phagocytic activity in diabetics which correlated with fasting blood sugar and glycosylated hemoglobin levels. This reversed with improvement in metabolic control.[42] Patients with diabetes are at an increased risk of developing pneumonia, TB, and fungal infections. Diabetes mellitus is a risk factor for developing mucormycosis. An air crescent sign is a risk factor for hemoptysis. Diagnosis is usually established from bronchoscopic samples or FNAC. The largest number of infections in the world is reported from India and diabetes mellitus is the most common risk factor. Treatment should include surgery with antifungals, where feasible.[7,43]

Approach to Patient with Suspected Pulmonary Infection

Any patient who is immunocompromised and has pulmonary infiltrates with or without constitutional symptoms needs to be evaluated for potential infections

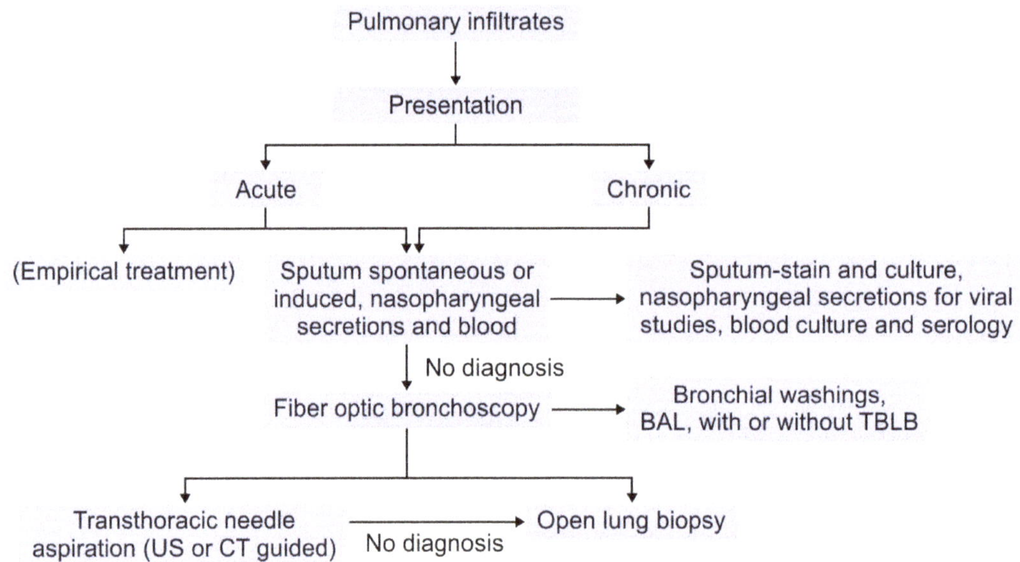

BAL, bronchoalveolar lavage; TBLB, transbronchial lung biopsy; US, ultrasound; CT, computed tomography.

Figure 2: Algorithm for evaluation of suspected lung infection in an immunocompromised host.

(Figure 2). If it is an acute presentation empirical treatment as determined by the causative organisms in the hospital or the community, it should be started while the evaluation for the causative organism is done. Systematic evaluation using noninvasive and invasive testing will give a definite etiological diagnosis in more than 80% of such episodes in immunocompromised patients and result in change in management in over 40% of patients.[31,33]

All patients should have blood samples drawn for cultures and serology. Culture should include bacteria and fungi, and serology includes *S. pneumoniae*, *Aspergillus*, and *Chlamydia pneumoniae*. If viral infections are a possibility and the facility is available, nasopharyngeal samples should be collected and immunofluorescent staining should be done to look for viral antigens (influenza viruses, respiratory syncytial virus, herpes simplex virus, etc.). Sputum spontaneous or induced should also be collected. A Gram stain to confirm the sample is adequate and stained for acid-fast bacili using Ziehl-Neelsen stain, *P. jirovicii* using Gomori, and Giemsa for fungus. Pearl's stain for hemosiderin laden macrophages should also be done in those with diffuse lung infiltrates as pulmonary hemorrhage is an important differential diagnosis. Bacterial, fungal, and mycobacterial cultures should be done on the obtained sample. Urine for pneumococcal antigen and legionella antigen should also been done.[33]

If there is no definite diagnosis and the patient has not responded to empirical treatment a bronchoscopy should be done and bronchial washings and lavage from the segment of interest should be taken. In the event of diffuse lung disease, lavage is done from the middle lobe or lingular lobe. Uncontrolled hypoxemia and thrombocytopenia less than $50 \times 10^6/\mu L$ are contraindications. A protected specimen brush can also be taken but has not shown to significantly improve the diagnostic yield over that obtained by bronchial washings, brushing, and BAL. The samples should be sent for staining and cultures as done for sputum. A transbronchial lung biopsy could be considered in those where PJP or TB are possibilities. It is also useful in confirming fungal infection by demonstrating tissue invasion.[31-33] Transthoracic FNAC should be considered if no diagnosis has been reached after bronchoscopy. It can be done using ultrasound or CT guidance. Computed tomography has the advantage that it can be done at the bedside. Two to three passes using a 22 G needle is done and the samples are smeared and stained as for sputum. Cultures should also be done and include bacterial, fungal, and mycobacterial.[44] In a retrospective study of 42 patients who had undergone FNAC, only 3 were inconclusive and there were no complications. This procedure is particularly useful for those lesions abutting the chest wall.[45]

PREVENTION

Some steps can be taken to decrease the incidence of infections in the immunocompromised patients. The simplest is to avoid exposure to respiratory pathogens particularly at the height of immunosuppression. Patients should consider simple measures like avoiding meeting people who are infected, avoiding travel to areas which are endemic to specific infections like fungi and wash hands. In areas which are endemic for TB, identifying and treating latent TB is an important step. Vaccination where possible should be given against seasonal influenza and pneumococcus. Vaccinating the immediate household contacts may also be useful. In those at high risk to develop *P. jirovicii*, chemoprophylaxis may be appropriate.[46]

CONCLUSION

Pulmonary infections in the immunocompromised patients are an important cause for morbidity and mortality. An understanding of the immunological defect and how it predisposes to infections with specific organisms is important. The population of immunocompromised has widened with the widespread use of immunosuppression and the epidemic of diabetes. Radiology and bronchoscopy are useful in helping establish the diagnosis. Outcomes are dependent on specific diagnosis and appropriate treatment.

Editor's Comment

Immunocompromised patients are more prone to infections and pneumonia is one of the most common infections in them. An immunocompromised patient is susceptible to not only infections with virulent organisms but also less virulent organisms to which a person with normal immunity is unlikely to be susceptible. Symptoms and signs depend on the pathogen and on the conditions compromising the immune system. The diagnosis and identification of causative microorganisms of pneumonia are often difficult in immunocompromised patients. Early etiological diagnosis and prompt treatment in these patients is a big challenge. Certain factors such as type of immunosuppression, epidemiological exposure, the time frame of infection in relation to immunosuppression and the clinicoradiological presentations are important in deciding the likely pathogen. An understanding of the immunological defect and how it predisposes to infections with specific organisms is important. These patients can rapidly worsen and require an aggressive diagnostic approach and early targeted therapy.

Ravindran Chetambath

REFERENCES

1. Hughes WT. Pneumonia in the immunocompromised child. *Semin Respir Infect.* 1987;2:177-83.
2. Oh YW, Effmann EL, Godwin JD. Pulmonary infections in immunocompromised hosts: The importance of correlating the conventional radiologic appearance with the clinical setting. *Radiology.* 2000;217:647-56.
3. Rosenow EC, Wilson WR, Cockerill FR. Pulmonary disease in the immunocompromised host. *Mayo Clin Proc.* 1985;60:473-87.
4. Tanakaya. Immunosuppressive mechanisms in diabetes mellitus. *Nihon Rinsho.* 2008;66:2233-37.
5. Agarwal AK, Gupta G, Marskole P, et al. A study of patients suffering from TB and TB diabetes co morbidity in RNTCP of northern MP, India. *Indian J Endocr Metab.* 2017;4:570-76.
6. Owiti P, Keter AD, Harries S, et al. Diabetes and pre-diabetes in TB in western Kenya using point-of-care glycated hemoglobin. *Public Health Action.* 2017;7:147-54.
7. Lee FY, Mossad SB, Adal KA. Pulmonary mucormycosis, the last 30 years. *Arch Intern Med.* 1999;159: 1301-309.
8. Ahuja J, Kanne J. Thoracic infections in immunocompromised patients. *Radiol Clin N Am.* 2014;52:121-36.
9. Kumar A, Daniel R, Wood KW, et al. Duration of hypotension before initiation of effective antimicrobial therapy is the critical determinant of survival in human septic shock. *Crit Care Med.* 2006;34:1589-96.
10. Redente EF, Jakubzick CV, Martin TR, et al. Innate immunity in Murray & Nadel's Text Book of respiratory Diseases. Elsevier Saunders; 2016. pp. 184-205.
11. Fontenot A, Simonian PL Adaptive immunity, Murray & Nadel's Text Book of Respiratory Medicine, 6th ed. Elsevier Saunders; 2016. pp. 206-23.
12. Buckley RH. Immunodeficiency diseases. *JAMA.* 1987;258:2841-50.
13. Malech HL, Gallin JI. Current concepts in immunology, neutrophils in human diseases. *N Engl J Med.* 1987;317:687-94.

14. Williams JL, Markowitz RI, Capitanio MA, et al. Immune deficiency syndromes. *Semin Roentgenol.* 1975;10: 83-89.
15. Roitt IM, Brostoff J, Male DK. Immunology, 4th ed. Barcelona, Spain: Mosby. 1996;9:1-15.
16. Ross SC, Densen P. Complement deficiency states and infection. *Medicine.* 1984;63:243-73.
17. Lithike W. Immunological impairment and susceptibility to infection after splenectomy. *JAMA.* 1976;236: 1376-77.
18. Gerson SL, Talbot GH, Hurwitz S, et al. Prolonged granulocytopenia: The major risk factor for invasive aspergillosis in patients with acute leukemia. *Ann Intern Med.* 1984;100:345-51.
19. Rubin RH, Wolfson JS, Cosimi AB, et al. Infection in the renal transplant recipient. *Am J Med.* 1981;70: 405-411.
20. Randhwa PS, Yousem SA. Epstein-Bar virus associated lymphoproliferative disease in a heart-lung allograft. *Transplantation.* 1990;49:126-130.
21. Rubin RH, Ferrao MJ. Understanding and diagnosisng infectious complications in the immunocompromised host. *Hematol Oncol Clin North Am.* 1993;7:795-812.
22. John GT, Shankar V, Abraham AM, et al. Risk factors for post-transplant tuberculosis. *Kidney Int.* 2001;60:1148-53.
23. Reynolds JH, Banerjee AK. Imaging pneumonia in immunocompetent and immunocompromised individuals. *Curr Opin Pulm Med.* 2012;18:194-201.
24. Muder RR, Yu VL, Parry MF. The radiologic manifestations of legionella pneumonia. *Semin Respir Infect.* 1988;2:242-54.
25. Pande A, Guharoy D. A case of pulmonary tuberculosis presenting as multiple nodular opacities on chest x-ray. *J Family Med Prim Care.* 2012;1:155-56.
26. Kuhlman JE, Fishman EK, Burch PA, et al. CT of invasive pulmonary aspergillosis. *Am J Roentgenol.* 1988;150:1015-20.
27. Demirkazik FB, Akin A, Omrum U, et al. CT findings in immunocompromised patients with pulmonary infections. *Diagn Interv Radiol.* 2008;14:75-82.
28. Moon JH, Kim EA, Lee KS, et al. Cytomegalovirus pneumonia: High resolution CT findings in ten non-AIDS immunocompromised patients. *Korean J Radiol.* 2000;1:73-78.
29. Chong S, Kim TS, Cho EY. Herpes simplex virus pneumonia: high-resolution CT findings. *Br J Radiol.* 2010;83:585-89.
30. Crawford SW. Non-infectious lung disease in immunocompromised host. *Respiration.* 1999;66:385-95.
31. Baselskin VS, Wundeink RG. Bronchoscopic diagnosis of pneumonia. *Clin Microbiol Rev.* 1994;7:553-58.
32. Stover DE, Zaman MB, Haidu SI, et al. Bronchoalveolar lavage in the diagnosis of diffuse pulmonary infiltrates in the immunocompromised host. *Ann Intern Med.* 1984;101:1-7.
33. Rano A, Augusti C, Jimenez P, et al. Pulmonary infiltrates in non-HIV immunocompromised patients: A diagnostic approach using non-invasive and bronchoscopic procedures. *Thorax.* 2001;56:379-87.
34. Lazarous DG, O'Donnell AE. Pulmonary infections in the HIV infected patient in the era of highly active antiretroviral therapy: an update. *Curr Infect Dis Rep.* 2007;9:228-32.
35. Ghate M, Deshpande S, Tripathy S, et al. Incidence of common opportunistic infections in HIV-infected individuals in Pune India; analysis by stage of immunosuppression represented by CD4 counts. *Int Infect Dis.* 2009;13:e1-8.
36. Patel AK, Thakarar SJ, Ghanchi, FD. Clinical and laboratory profile of patients with TB/HIV coinfection in a series of 50 patients. *Lung India.* 2011;28:93-96.
37. Wallis RS, Broder MS, Wong JY, et al. Granulomatous infectious diseases associated with tumor necrosis factor antagonists. *Clin Inf Dis.* 2004;38:1261-65.
38. Wallis RS, Schluger NW. Pulmonary infectious complications of tumor necrosis factor blockade. *Infect Dis Clin North Am.* 201;24:681-92.
39. Rostaing L, Malvezzi P. Steroid based therapy and risk of infectious complications. *PLos Med.* 2016;13(5): e1002025.

40. Stuck A, Minder CE, Frey FJ. Risk of infectious complication in patients taking glucocorticoids. *Clin Infect Dis.* 1989;11:954-63.
41. Fardet L, Peterson I, Nazareth I. Common infections prescribed systemic glucocorticoids in primary care: A population-based cohort study. *PLoS Med.* 2016;13(5):e1002024.
42. Lecube A, Pachon G, Petriz J, et al. Phagocytic activity is impaired in type 2 diabetes mellitus and increases after metabolic control. *PLoS One.* 2011;6(8):e23366.
43. Chakrabarti A, Chatterjee SS, Shivaprakash MR. Overview of opportunistic fungal infections in India. *Jap J Med Mycol.* 2008;49:165-72.
44. Corcoran JP, Tazi-Mezalek R, Maldonado F, et al. State of the art thoracic ultrasound: Interventions and therapeutics. *Thorax.* 2017;72:840-49.
45. Sharma S, Gupta P, Gupta N, et al. Pulmonary infections in immunocompromised patients: The role of image-guided fine needle aspiration cytology. *Cytopathology.* 2017;28:46-54.
46. Rubin LG, Levin MJ, Ljungman P, et al. 2013 IDSA clinical practice guideline for vaccination of the immunocompromised host. *Clin Infect Dis.* 2013;58:e44-e100.

World Clin Pulm Crit Care Med. 2019;6(1):121-34.

Atypical Pneumonias

Sanjeev Nair MD

Department of Pulmonary Medicine, Government Medical College
Thiruvananthapuram, Kerela, India

ABSTRACT

Atypical pneumonias include a group of pneumonias where the sputum examination and routine cultures do not reveal a predominantly bacterial etiology. Large number of agents has been implicated as the causative organisms in atypical pneumonias. The common ones among them are *Mycoplasma pneumoniae*, *Legionella pneumophila*, and *Chlamydophila pneumoniae*. A significant proportion of community-acquired pneumonias are caused by atypical organisms (ranging from 20 to 40% in various studies). The diagnosis and treatment of these pneumonias is different from pneumonias caused by organisms like *Streptococcus pneumoniae* and is often challenging.

INTRODUCTION

The term "atypical pneumonia" was historically used to describe those pneumonias which were caused by organisms other than *Streptococcus pneumoniae* and influenza virus. The pneumonias caused by such atypical organisms are called atypical because the clinical presentation, the radiological features, and antibiotics needed for treatment are different than those normally used for pneumococcal pneumonia. While the common organisms causing atypical pneumonias include *Mycoplasma pneumoniae*, *Legionella pneumophila*, and *Chlamydophila pneumoniae*, various authors list a large variety of bacteria and viruses as causative organisms of atypical pneumonias. This article discusses the epidemiology, etiopathogenesis, diagnosis, and treatment of atypical pneumonias, focusing primarily on the organisms mentioned above (Table 1).

Email: drsanjeevnair@gmail.com

Table 1: Organisms Listed as Cause of Atypical Pneumonias in Various Studies

Common organisms	Rare organisms		
	Bacteria	**Viruses**	**Fungi**
Mycoplasma pneumoniae	*Chlamydophila psittaci*	Respiratory syncytial virus	*Histoplasma*
Chlamydophila pneumoniae	*Bacillus anthracis*	Influenza virus	*Blastomyces*
Legionella pneumophila	*Francisella tularensis*	Parainfluenza virus	*Coccidioides*
	Yersinia pestis	Adenovirus	*Pneumocystis*
	Coxiella burnetii	Epstein–Barr virus	
		Cytomegalovirus	
		Hantavirus	

HISTORY

Historically atypical pneumonias were those which were not detectable by Gram stain or standard culture techniques. This term was initially used for viral pneumonias to differentiate them from bacterial pneumonias. The term has also been used to differentiate pneumonias caused by organisms other than *Streptococcus pneumoniae* and influenza virus. The patients with atypical pneumonias had more of constitutional symptoms as compared to the patients with pneumococcal pneumonias. In the 1930s and 1940s, many case series were reported describing cases with atypical pneumonia and some authors suggested that atypical pneumonias were caused by a virus which could be similar to the psittacosis virus. However, in 1942 Eaton demonstrated the presence of an organism which was very small, like a virus, which was called the Eaton agent. It was only in the 1960s that this was determined to be a bacterium, *Mycoplasma pneumonia* and found to be responsible for causing pneumonia in humans. Extensive experiments were done with respect to atypical pneumonias during the Second World War as this became a major problem for the US army.[1]

In the meantime, advances were also made in the diagnosis of atypical pneumonias like development of cold agglutinins in 1943 and development of a technique for fluorescent sustainable antibodies in 1957. In the 1960s, the Eaton agent was studied better and tissue culture-based techniques were developed and later cell-free media was used for the culture.

EPIDEMIOLOGY

Atypical pneumonias are not uncommon; however there is considerable variation in their proportion in various studies which try to determine the proportion of pneumonias caused by atypical organisms among all pneumonias (Table 2). These studies are hampered by the difficulty in growing the organisms as well as the fact that most pneumonias are treated empirically without an attempt to identify the causative organisms.

A meta-analysis on atypical pneumonias including data from 32 countries showed that the overall prevalence of *Mycoplasma pneumoniae*, *Legionella pneumophila*, and *Chlamydophila pneumonia* in patients with community-acquired pneumonias (CAP) was 10.1% (95% CI 7.1–13.1%), 2.8% (95% CI 2.1–3.6%), and 3.5% (95% CI 2.2–4.9%), respectively.[2]

A study was conducted on 1,374 subjects with pneumonia in eight Southeast Asian countries using serology, polymerase chain reaction (PCR), Enzyme-linked immunosorbent assay (ELISA) and urinary antigen for diagnosis. When serology alone was considered proportion of *Mycoplasma pneumoniae, Legionella pneumophila*, and *Chlamydophila pneumoniae* as the causative organism was 9.4%, 6.2%, and 4.3%, respectively. When serology was combined with ELISA and PCR, the proportions became 12.2%, 6.6% and 4.7%, respectively.[3] There are very few reports from India studying the proportions of atypical pneumonias, with most looking at biased samples in tertiary care hospitals and limited by small sample size. Proportions of atypical pneumonias in some recent studies are listed in table 2.

Mycoplasma pneumoniae is transmitted by person-to-person contact and spreads slowly, mostly within closed populations. Mini outbreaks of *Mycoplasma pneumoniae* do occur in schools and military camps but are often not recognized due to the long incubation period. *Legionella* infection is often seasonal, in summers, associated with the use of contaminated air conditioners or pooled water, particularly that which involves heating or cooling, such as condensers, cooling towers, respiratory therapy equipment, showers, water faucets and whirlpools. *Chlamydia pneumoniae* infection may be common in the population, it was seen that 50% of adults in the United States and 75% of elderly people had detectable antibodies to this bacteria[9].

Some of the other organisms listed as causative organisms for atypical pneumonias include some zoonotic organisms and these can be diagnosed on the basis of epidemiological clues, by eliciting the history of exposures which could lead to the infection. These include *Chlamydia psittaci*, which causes psittacosis, for which a history of exposure to birds like parrots and parakeets is an important clue. *Francisella tularensis*, which causes tularemia, is spread by exposure to tissues of infected animals, particularly rabbits, bite by cats, coyote or deer fly and through aerosols. *Coxiella burnetii*, which causes Q fever, is transmitted from aerosols from placenta and birth fluids of infected livestock like wild rabbits or cats.

Table 2: Proportions of Common Organisms Causing Atypical Pneumonias among Patients with Community-acquired Pneumonia (CAP)[2-8]

Country	Year	First Author	Patient group included	Number of subjects with CAP in the study	Proportion of organisms among patients with CAP		
					M. pneumoniae	*C. pneumoniae*	*L. pneumophila*
Eight Asian countries	2001-02	Yun-Fong	Patients with CAP presenting to medical centers	1374	12.20%	4.70%	6.60%
Thirty two high income countries	1998 2012	Christian Marchello	Meta-analysis—CAP, inpatient and outpatient	NA	10.10%	3.50%	2.80%
China	2003 2004	Youning Liu	CAP—non-severe and severe	610	13.40%	4.80%	2.80%
China	2011 2013	Keping Chen	Children with CAP	1204	40.78%	0.33%	0.91%
Twenty one countries	1996 2004	Arnold FW	Laboratory database	4337	12%	7%	5%
Netherlands	2007 2010	Van Gageldonk-Lafeber AB	CAP reaching emergency room of general hospital	339	5.90%	0.60%	2.10%
Spain	2006 2007	Alberto Capelastegui	Population based CAP patients	700	15.90%	9.49%	4.36%

Other organisms causing atypical pneumonias, including viruses and some bacteria, can be suspected on epidemiological clues by the fact that they occur as local or widespread epidemics, and often based on the geographical distribution.

Risk classification scores are used to predict prognosis in atypical pneumonias as in other CAPs. Various studies have looked into the risk factors for mortality in atypical pneumonias. A study by Miyashita et al. showed that higher score on pneumonia severity index, higher A-DROP (a scoring system for prognosticating pneumonia, the parameters measured are age, dehydration, respiration, disorientation, and blood pressure) severity and lower serum albumin are associated with higher mortality in patients with atypical pneumonia.[10]

ETIOPATHOGENESIS

The three common pathogens causing atypical pneumonias are *Mycoplasma pneumoniae, Chlamydophila pneumoniae,* and *Legionella pneumophila.* Mycoplasmas are among the smallest prokaryotic microbes present in nature and are wall-less, malleable organisms. It has a small cell size, 1–2 mm long and 0.1–0.2 mm wide and hence, cannot be detected by light microscopy. The colonies are also small and may have to be visualized through a stereomicroscope. *Chlamydophila pneumoniae* is an obligate intracellular bacterium which was first recognized as a respiratory pathogen only in 1986. *Legionella pneumophila* is an intracellular, gram-negative, and aerobic bacillus that replicates in the respiratory monocytic cells. Even though these are the common organisms implicated in atypical pneumonia, other organisms such as *Chlamydia psittaci*, *Francisella tularensis*, and *Coxiella burnetii*, certain respiratory viruses and fungi are also considered as etiological agents for atypical pneumonia.

Mycoplasma pneumoniae has an attachment organelle which is important for reproduction as well as host cellular interaction. There are cytoskeletal proteins in and around this organelle which facilitate attachment as well as motility. Once it is attached to the host cells, the pathological process begins. The bacteria produces hydrogen peroxide by metabolizing glycerol which causes injury to the epithelial cells as well as the cilia; and also denaturation of hemoglobin in erythrocytes and lipid peroxidation, eventually leading to cell lysis. A toxin called the community-acquired respiratory distress syndrome toxin is also produced and causes similar destruction. The bacteria through direct action and through interaction with cells results in the production of various cytokines and recruitment of immune cells. Some of the key receptors include the toll-like receptor-2 (TLR-2), TLR-4, and intracellular adhesions molecule receptor. Cell mediated immunity, particularly the alveolar macrophages, play the key role in the immune defense mechanism. This can protect the host but may also produce an allergy like immune inflammation of the lung. *Mycoplasma pneumoniae* does not have the ability to synthesize amino acids, fatty acids, etc. due to its small genome, but after permanent adherence to the respiratory epithelium, the organism extends microtubules into the host cells, enabling consumption of various nutrients and oxygen from the host cells, resulting in nutrient depletion and injury. While *Mycoplasma pneumoniae* is generally considered as an extracellular parasite, it can also invade and damage host cells. It has been shown to invade nonphagocytes and survive in them for often more than 6 months.[11] The varying clinical and radiological patterns of *Mycoplasma pneumoniae* are determined by the immune reaction against the bacteria. The bacteria cannot live in a free form and hence, needs to exist in asymptomatic hosts as a mucosal pathogen and spread by droplet infection.

Legionella, an intracellular organism, after phagocytosis by alveolar macrophages, gets enclosed in a vacuole. However, this vacuole, rather than undergoing the normal immune protective process of fusing with a lysosome and degradation, becomes a niche in which the *Legionella* can replicate. The bacteria use the host's cells, by modifying the cell protein synthesis, to produce the amino acids for its own metabolism.[12] The Icm/Dot (intracellular multiplication/defect in organelle trafficking genes) secretion system, guanosine triphosphatase activity, interactions between soluble N-ethylmaleimide-sensitive factor attachment protein receptors are some of the mechanisms by which the *Legionella* containing vacuole achieves its functional activity.

Chlamydia attaches to the cell wall and promote active ingestion. The elementary body is the metabolically inactive but infective form of the bacteria, which after infection transforms into the metabolically active reticulate bodies, which after about 48–72 hours later reorganize into the elementary bodies and are released by cell lysis. There is also another phenotype of the bacteria, which can remain inactive in the cells by secreting effector proteins which create an atmosphere in the cell conducive to the bacteria. This form of the bacteria is resistant to antibiotic action. The chlamydial type III secretory apparatus is a key factor in the virulence of the organism. In active infection, cell lysis occurs; however in chronic infection *Chlamydia* can inhibit cell apoptysis which is an immune defense mechanism. *Chlamydia pneumoniae* can infect variety of cells including alveolar epithelial cells, vascular endothelial cells and smooth muscle cells, fibroblasts, mononuclear cells, T-cells, dendritic cells, and glia cells. *Chlamydia pneumoniae* can also induce host cell activation and reprogramming through various receptor systems and cytokines, and is considered to have an important role in atherogenesis.[13]

CLINICAL FEATURES

Atypical pneumonias are associated with significant extrapulmonary manifestations. Mycoplasma pneumonia is often associated with headache, myalgia, sore throat, nonexudative pharyngitis, diarrhea, confusion, rash, and Raynaud's phenomenon. Skin rashes and bulliform myringitis may also be rarely seen as late features. Clinical course is usually mild; however, there could be complications like pleural effusion, empyema, pneumothorax, and acute respiratory distress syndrome.

Chlamydia pneumonia occurs usually in young adults as a mild sporadic pneumonia, but may be severe when it is a coinfection in persons infected with *Streptococcus pneumoniae*. It generally starts in an insidious manner, initially with fever, malaise, headache, and sore throat followed by a dry cough, which is often paroxysmal and worse at night. Chlamydial pneumonia usually presents with sore throat and headache, and then a nonproductive cough, often associated with low-grade fever that may persist for many months if not treated early. Most of the cases are mild; however, severe disease can occur and mortality rate has been estimated to be 9%. Death is usually associated with secondary infection and underlying comorbidities.[9]

Legionella pneumonia can present with varied symptoms including mild cough and low-grade or high-grade fever, altered mental status, and respiratory failure. Constitutional symptoms occur early in the disease, including headache, myalgia, anorexia, diarrhea, and malaise. Extrapulmonary manifestations include myocarditis, pericarditis, glomerulonephritis, pancreatitis, and peritonitis. The mortality rate in *Legionella* pneumonia is 14%.[9]

DIAGNOSIS

Diagnosis of atypical pneumonias is often a challenge, as these organisms are not readily identified on routine Gram smears and do not grow on routine cultures. A high degree of suspicion based on clinical clues, such as history of exposures, or epidemiological clues is needed to order the right investigations. Advances in molecular techniques have led to greater diagnostic yield in patients with atypical pneumonias.

Clinical and radiological clues may be important in the diagnosis of atypical pneumonias. The typical clinical features have been described above. There are many studies which have looked at diagnosis based on patient's characteristics and clinical features so as to differentiate atypical pneumonias from other pneumonias. While physician coverage for atypical bacteria was higher in higher age and patients with higher pneumonia severity index, a significant proportion of patients with atypical pneumonia did not get adequate antibiotic coverage. Hence, diagnosis of atypical pneumonia based on clinical grounds alone has its own limitations.[14] Masia et al. developed a predictive model for diagnosing atypical pneumonias including the variables such as age (<65 years), exposure to birds, normal white blood cell count, elevated aspartate aminotransferase level and lipopolysaccharide-binding protien serum level of less than 14 mg/L. This model with a score of more than three has a sensitivity of 35.2% and specificity of 93%.[15]

Chest X-ray may show patchy reticular or reticulonodular opacities or patchy consolidation, particularly in the perihilar region (Figure 1). Subsegmental atelectasis may be seen. Radiological findings are often more extensive than what is expected based on clinical features.

Computed tomography of the thorax may show focal ground-glass opacityin a lobular distribution, but may often be diffuse and bilateral and associated with bronchial wall thickening (Figure 2). There may also be evidence of pleural effusion. Diffuse ground glass nodules in a centrilobular pattern may be seen early in the course of the illness. Lobar consolidation is common in *Mycoplasma* pneumonia.

Laboratory Diagnosis

Cold agglutinins were used initially to diagnose *Mycoplasma pneumoniae* infections. However, low sensitivity and specificity made this test inferior to newer tests. Culture, done in an appropriate medium, is considered the gold standard for diagnosis; however, it is expensive, needs early specimen transfer, takes a lot of time and is available only in reference laboratories or academic hospitals. Media for culture is commercially available. The advantage is that whenever

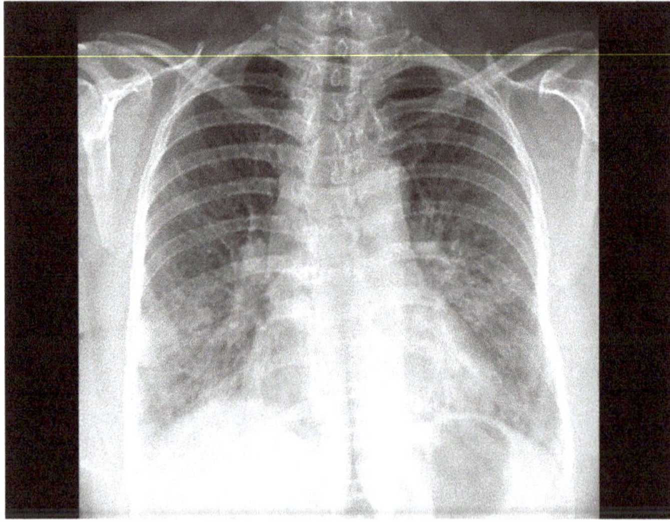

Figure 1: The X-ray chest posterior-anterior view showing diffuse infiltrates in a patient with *Mycoplasma pneumoniae* infection.

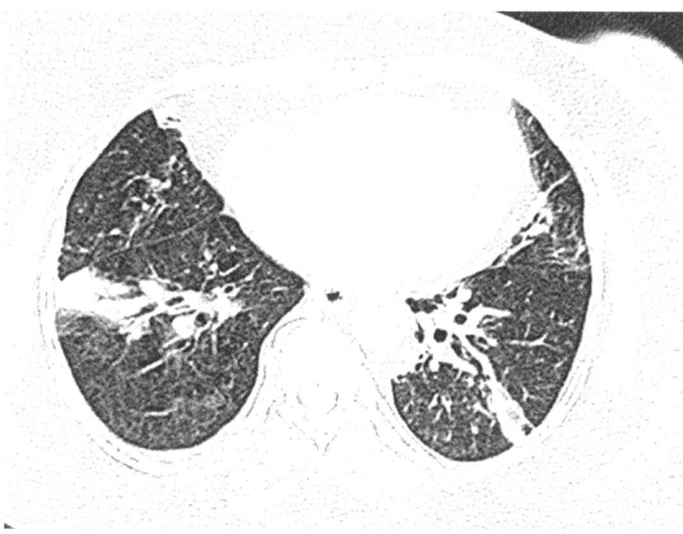

Figure 2: High resolution computed tomography thorax of a serologically confirmed *Mycoplasma pneumoniae* in a 35-year-old female presented with fever, cough, upper respiratory symptoms and hemolytic anemia.

Source: Arjun P, Thomas AV, Ameer KA. Can a Spurious Blood Result give a Clue to the Aetiological Diagnosis of Pneumonia? A Case Report. Kerala Medical Journal. 2016; 9(4):177-9.

positive, the test is 100% specific. Diagnosis of *Mycoplasma pneumoniae* infection is commonly performed by serological methods, like passive agglutination, compliment fixation, and ELISA. The ELISA is considered more sensitive than culture and has sensitivity similar to PCR, but is considered less sensitive than passive agglutination serology using paired sera. Faster results are obtained by detection of immunoglobulin M (IgM) antibodies; however, these may not be elevated in all patients. Other tests like complement fixation tests, indirect immunofluorescent assays, and particle agglutination assays have lower sensitivity and specificity. Combination of PCR with serology might provide optimal diagnosis. Molecular tests are available in the form of various commercially available kits for PCR as well as loop-mediated isothermal amplification assay. These tests provide rapid results and have high sensitivity and specificity; hence can be used to guide treatment decisions. The disadvantage is the cost and the need for expertise and equipment, as well as the fact that these have not been standardized.[16]

Culture is difficult in *Chlamydia pneumonia* too and is usually available only in reference laboratories; however, when available, it is useful in isolating organism in a wide variety of specimens and these specimens can be used for genotypic studies too. It has the disadvantage of low sensitivity and specificity and potential for contamination. Serological diagnosis can be done using commercially available kits and allow quantification; however, the disadvantages are low sensitivity and the test not being optimal for clinical decision making. Center for disease control (CDC-USA), considers micro-immunofluorescence as the serological method of choice. There are commercially available kits for molecular testing, with high sensitivity and specificity. The advantages are rapid detection and greater discriminatory power; hence, the test is useful for clinical decision making. The disadvantages are the cost and the need for expertise and equipment, as well as lack of standardization.[17]

The early tests developed for detection of *Legionella* included culture and direct fluorescent-antibody (DFA) assay. Development of tests with greater sensitivity and specificity has facilitated easier diagnosis. The tests currently used include bacterial culture (which is the gold standard), urinary antigen test (UAT), PCR and paired serology (either by indirect fluorescent-antibody assay or ELISA). The UAT has revolutionized the diagnosis of *Legionella* due to low cost, early results, ease of test, and commercial availability. The test is positive from 2 to 3 days from the start of symptoms and until 1–2 months of therapy.[18]

TREATMENT

Pneumonias are generally treated with empiric antibiotics as the results of culture and sensitivity testing take time and the isolation of etiological agent may not be possible in a large proportion of cases. The guideline-based treatment is discussed below.

While considering the treatment of known cases with atypical pneumonias, beta-lactams are not considered effective as *Mycoplasma pneumoniae* lacks a cell wall, and *Chlamydia pneumoniae* and *Legionella* species are intracellular organisms. Traditionally, erythromycin and tetracycline have been the drugs used for the treatment of atypical pneumonias. Macrolides (azithromycin and clarithromycin) are the drugs considered for the initial treatment for *M. pneumoniae, C. pneumoniae*, and *Legionella* species. Doxycycline is an alternative choice, which is less expensive, too. Fluoroquinolones also have excellent activity against *M. pneumoniae, C. pneumoniae*, and *Legionella* species.[9]

MANAGEMENT OF ATYPICAL PNEUMONIAS IN THE CONTEXT OF GUIDELINES FOR COMMUNITY-ACQUIRED PNEUMONIA

Diagnosis and treatment of pneumonias in clinical practice is generally based on current national and international guidelines. These are based on evidence, the common etiologies in that community, sensitivity pattern of organisms in that community and cost-effectiveness. Guidelines for CAPs do accept the fact that atypical pneumonias are not uncommon. However, testing for all the bacteria which cause atypical pneumonia is not practical due to low yield with most tests as well as lack of availability of the investigations and the high cost. Most guidelines recommend the testing for atypical pathogens only in specific clinical scenarios.

As per the IDSA/ATS (Infectious Diseases Society of America/American Thoracic Society) guidelines for CAP,[19] in the outpatient setting, routine testing for identifying an etiological agent is optional. For inpatients or those with severe pneumonia, a UAT for *Legionella* is recommended and if positive, a culture with special media for *Legionella* is recommended. Paired serology for atypical pathogens is not considered useful as the therapy would be completed before the time when second sample is due. The guidelines have pointed out that various types of PCR for atypical pneumonia are in clinical use; however, a high proportion of these do not satisfy the criteria of a validated test.

The National Institute for Health and Care Excellence (NICE) guidelines from United Kingdom do not recommend any microbiological tests in patients with low-severity CAP.[20] For patients with moderate or high severity CAP, *Legionella* UAT are recommended. The earlier British Thoracic Society (BTS) guidelines (2009), recommend UAT for *Legionella* for all cases of severe CAP and when positive, should be sent for culture. Culture for *Legionella* is also recommended for all invasive respiratory samples. The PCR for *Mycoplasma* and *Chlamydophila* is recommended in all cases of high severity CAP where there is strong suspicion. The guidelines point out that though, serological assay by complement fixation is the recommended serological test, it should be interpreted with caution in *Mycoplasma* and it cannot reliably detect acute infection due to *Chlamydia pneumoniae*.[21]

Indian guidelines for pneumonia[22] recommend that *Legionella* UAT is desirable in patients with severe CAP; however, investigations for atypical pathogens like *Mycoplasma, Chlamydia*, and viruses need not be routinely done.

Empiric antibiotic therapy is the norm for treating CAP. Early initiation of appropriate antibiotics is considered optimal for best outcomes. There is considerable difference between guidelines on what should be the antibiotic of choice. As per the IDSA/ATS guidelines for CAP,[19] the preferred antibiotics for outpatient management for patients with no comorbidities is a macrolide or doxycycline, whereas for CAP with comorbidities being managed as outpatient, the antibiotics of choice are a respiratory fluoroquinolone or beta-lactam plus a macrolide. All these options include antibiotics which are effective in atypical pneumonias. However, as per the BTS guidelines and NICE guidelines,[20,21] the drug of choice for a CAP being treated as outpatient is amoxicillin. For patients with moderate severity who are hospitalized the choice of antibiotic is amoxicillin plus a macrolide. In the Indian pneumonia guidelines[22] too, the drug of choice for a patient with pneumonia being managed as an outpatient is either amoxicillin or a macrolide. Both the NICE guidelines and the Indian guidelines recommend against fluoroquinolones in the outpatient setting for pneumonia.

These guidelines lead to a debate on whether coverage for atypical pneumonias is lacking in a significant proportion of patients with CAP. Various studies have looked at this aspect. Mills et al., did a meta-analysis[23] to compare beta-lactam antibiotics with antibiotics active against atypical pathogens in the management of CAP. The results of the meta-analysis did not support the need for antibiotics that possess specific activity against atypical pathogens in the initial management of adults with mild to moderate CAP. Similarly, Maimon et al. did a meta-analysis[24] to systematically compare outcomes between antibiotic classes in treating outpatient CAP, with regard to antibacterials active against atypical organisms, as well as between various antibacterial classes with similar atypical coverage. This meta-analysis did not find any demonstrable advantage of specific antibacterial agents for mild CAP in relatively healthy outpatients and the need for coverage of atypical pathogens was not apparent. Shefet et al. did a similar meta-analysis[25] to assess the efficacy of empirical coverage of atypical pathogens in terms of mortality, clinical and bacteriological success. This meta-analysis also showed no benefit of survival or clinical efficacy with empirical antibiotic coverage of atypical pathogens in hospitalized patients with CAP. From these studies, we can conclude that the choice of initial empiric antibiotics in various guidelines would not make a significant difference in outcomes in patients with atypical pneumonia.

CONCLUSION

Pneumonias due to atypical organisms are not uncommon. These account for 20–40% of CAP in various studies. The diagnosis of these infections is not easy; however, advances in diagnostics such as the availability of PCR or UAT have made the diagnosis quicker and easier, albeit with a significant cost. Most guidelines for CAP do not recommend routine testing for these organisms except for the UAT for *Legionella*. While, the antibiotics to which these organisms respond include macrolides, doxycycline, and fluoroquinolones, not all guidelines use these antibiotics as first choice empiric antibiotic for the treatment of CAP. However, various studies have shown that coverage for atypical organisms in the initial empiric treatment for CAP may not really make a significant difference in outcome. Clinical and epidemiological clues have to be kept in mind so as to suspect these organisms and in making a diagnosis. More studies on the epidemiology and outcomes are needed with respect to atypical pneumonias from developing countries like India so as to guide the local guidelines for CAP.

Editor's Comment

Atypical pneumonia is often missed in routine clinical work-up unless there is high index of suspicion or epidemiological data in a particular community. The atypical clinical presentation compared to typical pneumonia, difficulty in identifying the organism by Gram stain or culture and failure to respond to routine antibiotics are challenges to the treating physician. Atypical pneumonia spreads through close contact. Coughs and sneezes that contain the infectious pathogens pass through the air from person to person. Anyone who lives or works in an area where outbreaks of atypical pneumonia commonly occur may be more at-risk, as well. These places include school and college dormitories, nursing homes, and hospitals. As elaborated in this article three specific infectious bacteria cause the majority of atypical pneumonia cases. They are Mycoplasma pneumoniae, Chlamydophila pneumoniae, and Legionella pneumophila. Rapid diagnostic methods such as passive agglutination, compliment fixation, enzyme linked immunosorbent assay and polymerase chain reaction are now available for early detection of these diseases. All these entities respond well to macrolides or doxycycline. However, Mycoplasma strains and Legionella strains resistant to macrolides are being reported.

Ravindran Chetambath

REFERENCES

1. Saraya T. The history of *Mycoplasma pneumoniae* Pneumonia. *Front Microbiol.* 2016;7:364.
2. Marchello C, Dale AP, Thai TN, et al. Prevalence of atypical pathogens in patients with cough and community-acquired pneumonia: A meta-analysis. *Ann Fam Med.* 2016;14(6):552-66.
3. Ngeow YF, Suwanjutha S, Chantarojanasriri T, et al. An Asian study on the prevalence of atypical respiratory pathogens in community acquired pneumonia. *Int J Infect Dis.* 2005;9(3):144-53.
4. Liu Y, Chen M, Zhao T, et al. Causative agent distribution and antibiotic therapy assessment among adult patients with community acquired pneumonia in Chinese urban population. *BMC Infect Dis.* 2009;9:31.
5. Chen K, Jia R, Li L, et al. The aetiology of community associated pneumonia in children in Nanjing, China and aetiological patterns associated with age and season. *BMC Public Health.* 2015;15:113.
6. Arnold FW, Summersgill JT, LaJoie AS, et al. A worldwide perspective of atypical pathogens in community-acquired pneumonia. *Am J Respir Crit Care Med.* 2007;175:1086-93.
7. van Gageldonk-Lafeber AB, Wever PC, van der Lubben IM, et al., The aetiology of community-acquired pneumonia and implications for patient management. *Neth J Med.* 2013;71(8):418-25.
8. Capelastegui A, España PP, Bilbao A, et al. Etiology of community-acquired pneumonia in a population-based study: Link between etiology and patients characteristics, process-of-care, clinical evolution and outcomes. *BMC Infect Dis.* 2012;12:134.
9. Kristopher P, Thibodeau LC, Anthony J. Atypical pathogens and challenges in community-acquired pneumonia. *Am Fam Physician.* 2004;69(7):322-30.

10. Miyashita N, Kawai Y, Akaike H, et al. Clinical features and the role of atypical pathogens in nursing and healthcare-associated pneumonia (NHCAP): Differences between a teaching university hospital and a community hospital. *Intern Med.* 2012;51:585-94.
11. He J, Liu M, Ye Z, et al. Insights into the pathogenesis of *Mycoplasma pneumonia* (Review). *Mol Med Rep.* 2016;14(5):4030-6.
12. Price CT, Richards AM, Abu Kwaik Y. Nutrient generation and retrieval from the host cell cytosol by intra-vacuolar *Legionella pneumophila. Front in Cell Infect Microbiol.* 2014;4:111.
13. Kern JM, Maass V, Maass M. Molecular pathogenesis of chronic *Chlamydia pneumonia* infection: A brief overview. *Clin Microbiol Infect.* 2009;15:36-41.
14. Piso RJ, Arnold C, Bassetti S. Coverage of atypical pathogens for hospitalized patients with community-acquired pneumonia is not guided by clinical parameters. *Swiss Med Wkly.* 2013;143: w13870.
15. Masiá M, Gutiérrez F, Padilla S, et al. Clinical characterization of pneumonia caused by atypical pathogens combining classic and novel predictors. *Clin Microbiol Infect.* 2007;13(2):153-61.
16. Centre for disease control and prevention [Internet]. Mycoplasma pneumoniae infection Diagnostic methods; [cited July 06 2017]. Available from: https://www.cdc.gov/pneumonia/atypical/mycoplasma/hcp/diagnostic-methods.html
17. Centre for disease control and prevention [Internet]. Chlamydia pneumoniae infection. [cited July 06 2017]. Available from: https://www.cdc.gov/pneumonia/atypical/cpneumoniae/hcp/diagnostic.html
18. Mercante JW, Winchell JM. Current and Emerging Legionella Diagnostics for Laboratory and Outbreak Investigations. *Clin Microbiol Rev.* 2015;28(1):95-133.
19. Mandell LA, Wunderink RG, Anzueto A, et al. Infectious Diseases Society of America/American Thoracic Society Consensus Guidelines on the Management of Community-Acquired Pneumonia in Adults. *Clinl Infect Dis.* 2007;44:S27-72.
20. National Institute for Health and Care Excellence (NICE) [Internet]. Pneumonia in adults: Diagnosis and management: Clinical guideline [CG191]; December 2014 [cited 2017 July 07]. Available from: https://www.nice.org.uk/guidance/cg191
21. WS Lim, SV Baudouin, RC George, et al. British Thoracic Society guidelines for the management of community acquired pneumonia in adults: Update 2009. *Thorax.* 2009;64(Suppl III):iii1-55.
22. Gupta D, Agarwal R, Aggarwal AN, et al. Guidelines for diagnosis and management of community and hospital acquired pneumonia in adults: Joint ICS/NCCP (I) Recommendations. *Indian J Chest Dis Allied Sci.* 2012;54:267-81.
23. Mills GD, Oehley MR, Arrol B. Effectiveness of β-lactam antibiotics compared with antibiotics active against atypical pathogens in non-severe community acquired pneumonia: Meta-analysis. *BMJ.* 2005; 330(7489):456.
24. Maimon N, Nopmaneejumruslers C, Marras TK. Antibacterial class is not obviously important in outpatient pneumonia: A meta-analysis. *Eur Respir J.* 2008;31:1068-76.
25. Shefet D, Robenshtok E, Paul M, et al. Empirical atypical coverage for inpatients with community-acquired pneumonia-systematic review of randomized controlled trials. *Arch Intern Med.* 2005;165:1992-2000.

World Clin Pulm Crit Care Med. 2019;6(1):135-45.

Viral Pneumonia

[1,*]Ravindran Chetambath MD DTCD FRCP MBA,
[2]Safreena M Nambipunnilath MD

[1]Department of Pulmonary Medicine, DM Wayanad Institute of Medical Sciences
Wayanad, Kerala, India
[2]Department of Pulmonary Medicine, Institute of Chest Diseases, Government Medical College
Kozhikode, Kerala, India

ABSTRACT

Viral infection is present in a high proportion of community-acquired pneumonia cases despite the obvious fact that the actual incidence is underestimated. Molecular diagnostic tests can aid in establishing a definitive diagnosis of viral pneumonias. Early initiation of treatment with specific antiviral drugs can reduce the mortality and morbidity in influenza pneumonia. Supportive treatment is recommended for most of the other viral pneumonias. Identification of a viral etiology could limit the inappropriate use of antibiotics. The growing epidemiological significance of viral pneumonias warrants further research for the development of effective antiviral drugs and newer vaccines. This article summarizes the common viral infections of the lower respiratory tract highlighting the newer diagnostic methods and management options.

INTRODUCTION

Respiratory viruses have been recently recognized as a potential cause of pneumonia in adults.[1] It has been consistently demonstrated through many studies that viruses are the second most common etiologic cause for community-acquired pneumonia (CAP), accounting for 13–50% of diagnosed cases.[2] Children and elderly are the most affected by viral pneumonias. Based on the atypical clinical and radiologic manifestations, viral pneumonia is included in the category of atypical pneumonias. This group includes viral pneumonias and the other atypical bacterial pneumonias. Clinical presentation of viral pneumonia are poor indicators

*Corresponding author
Email: crcalicut@gmail.com

of an etiological diagnosis[3] and may vary from a mild, self-limiting illness to a life-threatening disease depending on the virulence of the organism, age of the patient, and presence of other comorbidities. In immunocompromised patients, viral pneumonia may manifest as severe pneumonia resulting in hypoxemia and acute respiratory failure.

CLINICAL CLASSIFICATION

Viral pneumonia in adults can be divided into two groups: (i) viral pneumonia in otherwise normal hosts, and (ii) viral pneumonia in immunocompromised hosts.[4] Influenza virus type A is the most common virus followed by adenovirus and rhinovirus in immunocompetent adults. Immunocompromised hosts are susceptible to pneumonias caused by cytomegalovirus (CMV), herpes virus, measles virus, and adenovirus.

ETIOLOGY

- Influenza virus
- Respiratory syncytial virus
- Parainfluenza virus (PIV)
- Adenovirus
- Measles virus
- Hantavirus
- Herpes simplex virus
- Varicella-zoster virus
- Cytomegalovirus
- Epstein–Barr virus
- Newer emerging viruses such as human metapneumovirus, bocavirus, coronavirus, etc.

Influenza Pneumonia

Influenza virus infection usually involves the upper respiratory tract including the trachea and majorly, bronchi in children and young adults. However, elderly and immunocompromised persons are at increased risk for development of pneumonia. Type A and occasionally, type B influenza virus cause influenza virus pneumonia.[5] Although the pneumonia is usually mild, it can be overwhelming and fatal within 24 hours. In 2009, an outbreak of influenza caused by a novel influenza A (H1N1) virus was reported which spread rapidly to most parts of the world. From April 2009 to November 2009, a total of 30,533 confirmed cases were reported from various parts of India out of which 1,487 succumbed to the infection. This particularly affected the southern region with maximum cases being reported from Kerala. Number of cases reported in 2010 from the state was 3,250 out of which 137 patients succumbed to the illness.[6] In an observational study in a tertiary hospital in North Kerala, out of the 110 confirmed cases of H1N1 influenza, 72 were females which include 42 pregnant women. Total number of deaths in this group was 10 (9%) and pregnancy is not associated with increased mortality.[7]

Respiratory Syncytial Virus Pneumonia

Respiratory syncytial virus (RSV) is the most frequent cause of lower respiratory tract infection in infants and children and the second most common viral cause of pneumonia in adults. Patients with RSV pneumonia typically present with fever, rhinorrhea, nonproductive cough, and dyspnea. Wheezing occurs in approximately 20% of infants, 50% of older children, and 35% of older adults presenting to the outpatient departments.[8]

Parainfluenza Virus Pneumonia

Parainfluenza virus is another important cause of lower respiratory tract disease in children. The infection usually manifests as pneumonia and bronchiolitis in infants younger than 6 months. Parainfluenza virus pneumonia and bronchiolitis are caused primarily by the PIV-3 strain. The signs and symptoms include fever, coryza, cough, dyspnea, and wheezing.

Adenovirus Pneumonia

Adenovirus infection may manifest as pharyngitis, pharyngoconjunctivitis, laryngotracheobronchitis, bronchiolitis, or pneumonia. The adenovirus may also be involved in the pathogenesis of bronchiectasis.[9] Immunocompromised patients are more prone to develop severe pneumonia with adenovirus.

Measles Virus Pneumonia

Pulmonary disease from measles virus infection occurs mainly in two forms:

1. Primary measles virus pneumonia and secondary bacterial pneumonia
2. Atypical measles virus pneumonia.

Although measles virus can cause pneumonia in 3–4% of infected patients, the majority suffer from secondary bacterial infection. Measles virus pneumonia is more among pregnant women and patients with hematologic malignancy, acquired immunodeficiency syndrome (AIDS), or who are on immunosuppressive therapy.[10,11]

Hantavirus Pneumonia

Hantaviruses are lipid-enveloped, single-stranded ribonucleic acid viruses which cause a typical symptom complex called hemorrhagic fever with renal syndrome. Hantavirus also causes severe and fulminant pulmonary disease.[12] The organism is believed to be transmitted to humans by inhalation of dried rodent excreta associated with outdoor activities in rural areas. Hantavirus pulmonary syndrome characteristically manifest as acute respiratory distress syndrome (ARDS).

Herpes Simplex Virus Pneumonia

Herpes simplex virus affects patients who are immunocompromised or whose airways have been traumatized from intubation or smoke inhalation.[13] Infection spread to lower respiratory tract either by aspiration from oropharyngeal infection or through hematogenous spread in patients with sepsis.[14]

Varicella-zoster Virus Pneumonia

Varicella-zoster virus pneumonia is always a complication of disseminated varicella-zoster infection with mortality rates varying from 9 to 50%.[15] Varicella-zoster infection usually causes self-limited benign disease in children, where as in adults it leads to serious complications such as varicella-zoster virus pneumonia. Patients with lymphoma and immunocompromised status are particularly prone to develop this complication.

Cytomegalovirus Pneumonia

Cytomegalovirus cause severe symptomatic pulmonary disease such as severe necrotizing pneumonia in organ transplant recipients and AIDS patients. Cytopathogenic effects of CMV are believed to be the mechanism. Very high mortality is reported in CMV pneumonia.

Epstein–Barr Virus Pneumonia

Epstein–Barr virus causes infectious mononucleosis and pulmonary manifestation is relatively rare.[16] Infectious mononucleosis usually occurs in young adults aged 15–30 years and usually resolves over a period of weeks or months without any sequelae. Rarely, it is complicated by multiple system involvement including pneumonia.

Newer Emerging Viruses Causing Pneumonia

Human metapneumovirus (hMPV) may be the cause of a significant proportion of both upper and lower respiratory tract infection in infants, children, and adults. The results of several studies suggest that hMPV may account for about 10% of respiratory tract infections in which a common respiratory virus, such as respiratory syncytial virus, influenza or PIVs could not be detected. hMPV infection was associated with clinical diagnoses of pneumonia (36%), asthma exacerbations (23%), or acute bronchiolitis (10%).

Human bocavirus (HBoV) is another worldwide respiratory pathogen which is highly diverse, dispersed, recombination prone, and prevalent in endemic areas. HBoV-1 is found associated with lower respiratory infections in young children. HBoV infection presents with a variety of signs and symptoms which include rhinitis, pharyngitis, pneumonia, acute otitis media, and diarrhea.

Severe acute respiratory syndrome (SARS) is a serious form of pneumonia caused by a virus that was first identified in 2003. Infection with the SARS virus causes pneumonia, acute respiratory distress, and sometimes death. SARS is caused by a member of the coronavirus family of viruses and the 2003 epidemic started when the virus spread from small mammals in China.

A new strain of coronavirus has emerged in Saudi Arabia in 2012 causing Middle East respiratory syndrome (MERS). This novel coronavirus (MERS coronavirus or MERSCoV) can cause diseases ranging from common cold to SARS. Typical MERS symptoms include fever, cough and shortness of breath. Pneumonia is common, but not always present. Gastrointestinal symptoms, including diarrhea, have also been reported. Though the number of people affected is less, it has killed 65% of the affected patients and hence, raises concern among health workers.[17]

PATHOLOGY

Pathological manifestations of viral respiratory tract infections include tracheobronchitis, bronchiolitis, and pneumonia. The organisms usually replicate within the cells and cause histologic changes in the epithelium and adjacent interstitial tissue. In tracheobronchitis, airway walls are congested with cellular infiltration of mononuclear cells leading to degeneration and desquamation of the epithelial cells. Bronchiolitis causes mononuclear infiltrates, epithelial necrosis, and neutrophilic exudate in the lumen particularly in young children.[18] In pneumonia, lung adjacent to the terminal and respiratory bronchioles is initially involved, and extends throughout the lobule as the disease progresses. Severe, life-threatening progression may be seen in the elderly and immunocompromised patients.[19] In this stage, the lungs histologically resembles ARDS with diffuse alveolar damage due to interstitial lymphocyte infiltration, air-space hemorrhage, edema, type-2 cell hyperplasia, and hyaline membrane formation.[20]

CLINICAL FEATURES

The clinical manifestations (Table 1) in viral respiratory tract infections vary depending on the age of the patient, health status, and whether the infection is primary or secondary. Infants and young children with primary infections usually present with bronchiolitis or pneumonia, whereas older children and adults have mostly tracheobronchitis. They may develop pneumonia if they are elderly or immunocompromised.

DIAGNOSIS

Despite enhanced laboratory techniques such as viral culture, rapid antigen detection, and gene amplification, a confident diagnosis of viral pneumonia continues to be a challenge. The nonspecific nature of clinical characteristics and the extreme sensitivity of laboratory technique makes the diagnosis difficult, even when a viral agent is detected.

- Complete blood count: Leukocytosis is not marked in viral infections when compared to bacterial infections. Lymphocytes are the predominant cells. C-reactive protein is often elevated
- X-ray chest: Chest radiographs demonstrate normal findings or unilateral or patchy bilateral areas of consolidation (Figure 1), nodular opacities, and small

Table 1: Clinical Features of Viral Pneumonia

Symptoms	Signs
• Cough, mostly dry cough	• Tachypnea and/or dyspnea
• Fever, which may be mild or high	• Tachycardia or bradycardia
• Shaking chills	• Rhonchi
• Shortness of breath	• Crackles
• Other symptoms include:	• Sternal or intercostal retractions
○ Pleuritic chest pain	• Dullness to percussion
○ Confusion	• Decreased breath sounds
○ Excessive sweating	• Pleural friction rub
○ Headache	• Cyanosis
○ Loss of appetite	• Rash
○ Fatigue	• Respiratory distress

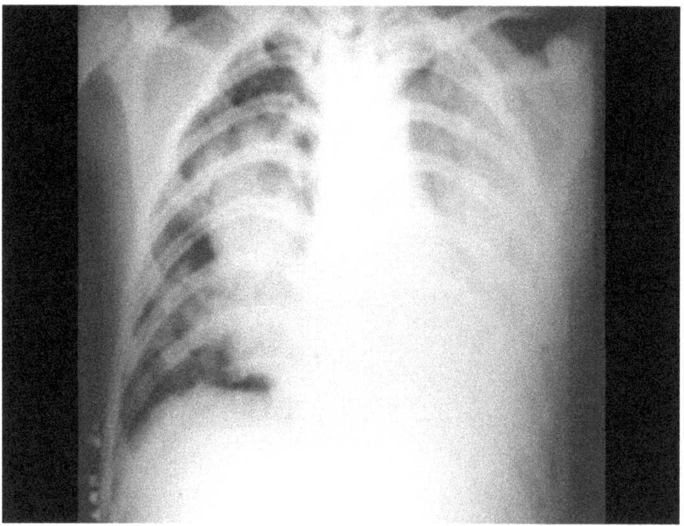

Figure 1: Rapidly progressing bilateral pneumonia in a case of H1N1 influenza infection.

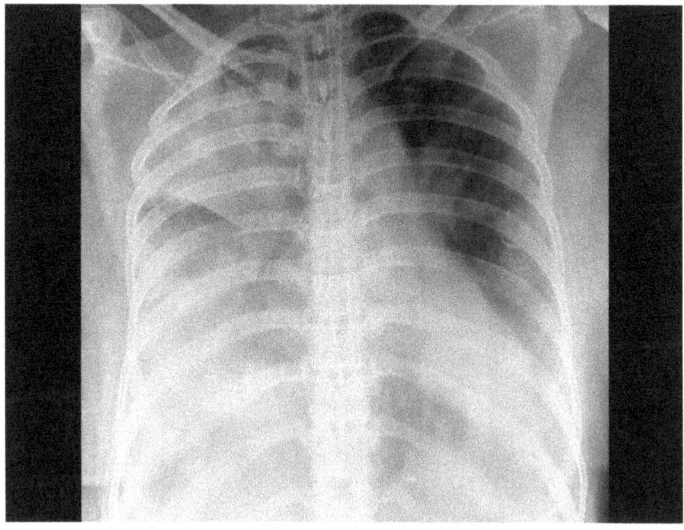

Figure 2: X-ray of a 53-year-old female with fever and breathlessness (throat swab positive for H1N1 influenza).

pleural effusions. Lobar consolidation is uncommon in patients with viral pneumonia. Patients may develop pneumonia with rapid progression to acute respiratory distress syndrome (Figure 2)[21]

- Computed tomography (CT) scan of the chest: Its findings include (i) parenchymal attenuation disturbances due to air trapping and hyperinflation associated with obstructive bronchiolitis;[18] (ii) ground-glass opacity and consolidation (Figure 3); (iii) nodules, micronodules, and tree-in-bud opacities; (iv) interlobular septal thickening; and (v) bronchial and/or bronchiolar wall thickening

- Throat and nasal swab tests: The laboratory diagnosis of viral respiratory tract infection is made by analysis of respiratory secretions. A nasal wash may provide best yield in healthy older children. Nasopharyngeal swab or throat swab may be usually done in acute infections. In intubated patients or who are immunocompromised, bronchoalveolar lavage should be obtained. Within 24 hours after admission, the homogenized samples were processed for antigen detection by indirect immunofluorescence assay (IFA), for isolation of viruses in cell culture and for detection of nucleic acids by two independent multiplex real-time polymerase chain reaction (RT-PCR)
- For IFA, the specimens are spotted onto glass slides and then dried and fixed in acetone. Monoclonal antibodies are used for detection of influenza A and B viruses, PIVs 1, 2, and 3, RSV, and adenovirus. The presence of viral antigen in respiratory cells is indicated by the appearance of characteristic intracellular apple-green fluorescence
- Viral culture: Specimens are inoculated into two human epithelial cells (Hep-2 and A-549) and into Madin-Darby canine kidney cells and incubated at 35°C during 3 weeks for primary viral isolation of influenza viruses, PIVs, RSV, and adenoviruses. Conventional cultures were examined twice weekly for the development of cytopathic effects. In cultures with positive results, virus was identified by staining with IFA

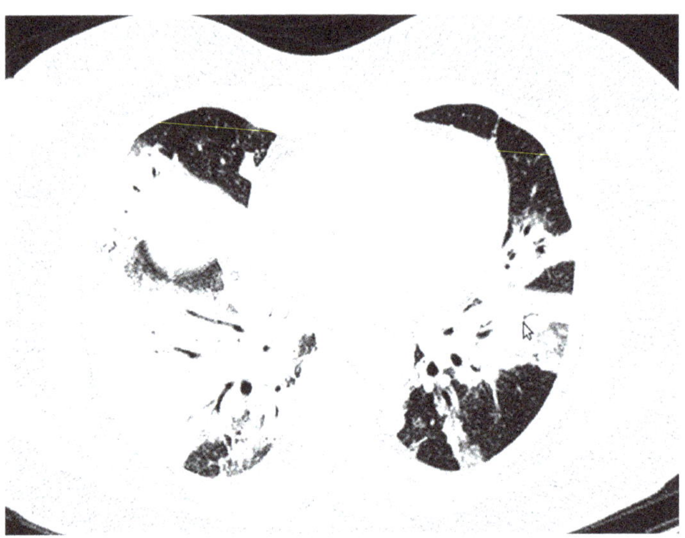

Figure 3: Computed tomography thorax showing bilateral consolidation (H1N1 influenza pneumonia).

- Rapid antigen assays: Assays utilizing antigen capture technology are the mainstay of diagnosis. These tests have relatively high sensitivity and specificity and can be performed in less than 30 minutes
- Blood cultures to check for viruses in the blood
- Polymerase chain reaction assay: Two independent multiplex reverse transcription nested RT-PCR assays are used to detect viral copies. Specific primers are used for influenza viruses types A, B, and C, RSV type A and B, adenovirus, PIVs 1, 2, 3, and 4, coronaviruses, and rhinoviruses[22]
- Open lung biopsy: Only done in very serious illnesses when the diagnosis cannot be made from other sources.

TREATMENT

Treatment should be initiated within 36 hours of the beginning of symptoms in influenza infection. Drugs available are adamantanes (amantadine and rimantadine) and neuraminidase inhibitors (oseltamivir and zanamivir). Antiviral therapy with neuraminidase inhibitors should be started empirically in all hospitalized patients, in whom influenza is suspected, including those with CAP. Zanamivir is available as powder for inhalation. Varicella pneumonia is almost always serious and is treated with acyclovir. Respiratory syncytial virus infection usually needs treatment for symptoms only. If serious infection is detected, it is to be treated with ribavirin. In PIV infection, treatment is mainly supportive, but aerosolized and oral ribavirin may be useful in reducing viral shedding and clinical improvement in immunocompromised patients. Cidofovir therapy has been associated with clinical improvement and increased survival in adenoviral infection, especially in transplant recipients.

PREVENTION

In situations where infection is suspected, the following precautions are important to prevent transmission.

- Wash the hands often, especially after blowing the nose, going to the bathroom, diapering a baby, and before eating or preparing food
- Avoid smoking as tobacco smoke will damage the mucosa and virus can easily enter the system
- Vaccines may help prevent pneumonia in children, the elderly, and people with diabetes, asthma, emphysema, human immunodeficiency virus, cancer, or other chronic conditions. Influenza vaccines are available and it must be given each year to protect against new virus strains
- Palivizumab is a humanized monoclonal antibody that is given to children below 2 years to prevent pneumonia caused by respiratory syncytial virus.

CONCLUSION

Viruses are the second most common etiologic cause for CAP. Viral pneumonias are included under atypical pneumonias because of the atypical clinical and radiological manifestations. Influenza virus type A, adenovirus, and rhinoviruses are the most frequently identified organisms causing pneumonia in immunocompetent adults. Newer emerging viruses like hMPV, HBoV, and MERSC are also recognized as causative agents for pneumonia. The clinical picture in viral pneumonia is nonspecific and ranges from a mild infection to life-threatening disease. The detection of virus or viral antigens in upper and lower respiratory samples is usually made based on culture and immunofluorescence microscopy. The use of real-time reverse-transcriptase PCR-based assays has improved the detection of respiratory viruses. Specific antiviral therapy is effective in influenza pneumonia. Annual vaccination is recommended to reduce the transmission of influenza viruses.

Editor's Comment

The incidence of viral pneumonias is likely to be high considering the highly infectious nature of most of the causative viruses. In spite of the advances in diagnostic tests such as the viral culture, rapid antigen detection, and gene amplification, a confident diagnosis of viral pneumonia is difficult to establish. They occur more often during extremes of age and other immune-suppressed conditions. Not uncommonly, viral pneumonias, especially influenza pneumonia occur in epidemic, or sometimes pandemic proportions. Viral pneumonias are frequently referred to as atypical pneumonias because of the nonspecific clinical and radiological manifestations. The clinical picture varies from a mild infection to life-threatening disease. It is important to initiate an early treatment to contain the disease complications and prevent mortality. Treatment is mostly supportive in nature while specific antiviral therapy is effective in influenza pneumonia.

Surinder K Jindal

REFERENCES

1. File TM. Community-acquired pneumonia. *Lancet.* 2003;362:1991-2001.
2. Jennings LC, Anderson TP, Beynon KA, et al. Incidence and characteristics of viral community-acquired pneumonia in adults. *Thorax.* 2008;63(1):42-8.
3. Ruiz M, Ewig S, Marcos MA, et al. Etiology of community acquired pneumonia in hospitalized patients: Impact of age, comorbidity and severity. *Am J Resp Crit Care Med.* 1999;160:397-405.
4. Sullivan CJ, Jordan MC. Diagnosis of viral pneumonia. *Semin Respir Infect.* 1988;3:148-61.

5. Nolan TF, Goodman RA, Hinman AR, et al. Morbidity and mortality associated with influenza B in the United States, 1979–1980: A report from the Centers for Disease Control. *J Infect Dis.* 1980;142:360-62.
6. Chetambath R. Resurgence of H1N1 Influenza in 2010 (Editorial). *Chest (India Edition).* 2010;2(4):195-99.
7. James PT, Sandeep BR, Santhosh PV, et al. A study to analyze the clinical profile and outcome of hospitalized patients with H1N1 and the factors influencing the outcome. *E R J.* 2011;38:4355-56.
8. Lee N, Lui GC, Wong KT, et al. High morbidity and mortality in adults hospitalized for respiratory syncytial virus infections. *Clin Infect Dis.* 2013;57:1069-73.
9. Bateman ED, Hayashi S, Kuwano K, et al. Latent adenoviral infection in follicular bronchiectasis. *Am J Respir Crit Care Med.* 1995;151:170-76.
10. Atmar RL, Englund JA, Hammill H. Complications of measles during pregnancy. *Clin Infect Dis.* 1992;14: 217-26.
11. Kaplan LJ, Daum RS, Smaron M, et al. Severe measles in immunocompromised patients. *JAMA.* 1992;267: 1237-41.
12. Butler JC, Peters CJ. Hantaviruses and hantavirus pulmonary syndrome. *Clin Infect Dis.* 1994;19:387-94.
13. Graham BS, Snell JD. Herpes simplex virus infection of the adult lower respiratory tract. *Medicine.* 1983;62:384-93.
14. Ramsey PG, Fife KH, Hackman RC, et al. Herpes simplex virus pneumonia: Clinical, virologic, and pathologic features in 20 patients. *Ann Intern Med.* 1982;97:813-20.
15. Nilsson A, Ortqvist A. Severe varicella pneumonia in adults in Stockholm County 1980-1989. *Scand J Infect Dis.* 1996;28:121-23.
16. Haller A, von Segesser L, Baumann PC, et al. Severe respiratory insufficiency complicating Epstein-Barr virus infection: Case report and review. *Clin Infect Dis.* 1995;21:206-9.
17. Chetambath R. Emerging Respiratory Viral Infections (Editorial). *Pulmon.* 2013; 15(1):6-8.
18. Galloway RW, Miller RS. Lung changes in the recent influenza epidemic. *Br J Radiol.* 1959;32:28-32.
19. Han BK, Son JA, Yoon HK, et al. Epidemic adenoviral lower respiratory tract infection in pediatric patients: Radiographic and clinical characteristics. *AJR Am J Roentgenol.* 1998;170:1077-80.
20. Tillett HE, Smith JW, Clifford RE. Excess morbidity and mortality associated with influenza in England and Wales. *Lancet.* 1980;1:793-95.
21. Yeldandi AV, Colby TV. Pathologic features of lung biopsy specimens from influenza pneumonia cases. *Hum Pathol.* 1994;25:47-53.
22. Cuchacovich R. Clinical applications of the polymerase chain reaction: An update. *Infect Dis Clin North Am.* 2006;20(4):735-58.

World Clin Pulm Crit Care Med. 2019;6(1):146-67.

Fungal Pneumonias

Raseela Karunakaran DTCD MD

Department of Pulmonary Medicine, Government TD Medical College
Alappuzha, Kerala, India

ABSTRACT

Bacteria were considered as the main cause of pneumonia worldwide. Nonbacterial pathogens such as fungi, virus, and parasites are also being detected as the cause of pulmonary infections. Various fungi cause serious lung infections and raise challenges in early diagnosis and management. The usual clinical, pathological, and roentgenological pictures are essentially the same for most of the pneumonias and separation into etiological entities must be accomplished by laboratory studies. Identification of demographic location for endemicity and high index of suspicion based on clinical presentation are important to establish a fungal etiology for pneumonia.

INTRODUCTION

Fungal pneumonias though considered rather uncommon earlier are being diagnosed with increasing frequency. This is attributed to the increasing number of susceptible population as a result of widespread use of drugs such as antibiotics, corticosteroids, immunosuppressants, use of devices, organ transplantation, and acquired immunodeficiency. Increasing number of fungal infections in the pulmonary and critical care units has significantly affected the health care costs in many countries. Mortality due to fungal infections is considered almost equal to that of tuberculosis and human immunodeficiency virus (HIV) disease. Many people at risk for and suffering from fungal diseases live in resource-limited settings, where diagnosis and treatment of these infections can be challenging.[1]

Email: raseeladr@yahoo.com

PATHOGENESIS

Fungi are ubiquitous organisms with saprophytic or parasitic existence.[2] As against the older concept, now it is clear that the lower respiratory tract of healthy people is not sterile, but comprises previously unappreciated complex microbial community termed as the lung microbiome.[3] The human lung microbiome is polymicrobial, which includes fungal community (mycobiome) along with bacteria and viruses. Most of the common fungi like *Candida*, *Aspergillus*, *Penicillium*, and *Cryptococcus* are seen in the lung mycobiome. The fungal biofilm formation contributes to increased drug tolerance and resistance to antifungal drugs.[4]

Pulmonary fungal pathogens are grouped into either primary pathogens or opportunistic pathogens. Primary fungal pathogens cause disease in immunocompetent hosts, e.g., *Histoplasma capsulatum*, *Coccidioides immitis*, *Paracoccidioides brasiliensis*, and *Blastomyces dermatitidis*. Opportunistic fungal pathogens cause disease in individuals with compromised immune system or in individuals with damaged epithelial barriers. This group include *Cryptococcus neoformans*, *Aspergillus fumigatus*, *Candida albicans*, *Pneumocystis jirovecii*, and *Rhizopus*.[5]

Pulmonary Aspergillosis

Aspergillus is a ubiquitous saprophytic fungus commonly isolated from both the outdoor and indoor environment including hospitals. Heat, moisture, and organic matters favor its growth. *Aspergillus fumigatus* is the most common pathogen. *A. terreus*, *A. niger*, and *A. flavus* are the other important pathogens causing disease in man. *Aspergillus* causes a variety of infections or allergic diseases in human hosts and the type of clinical disease depends on the host immune status and pulmonary structure.

Aspergillus-associated lung diseases are grouped into different types (Figure 1). In atopic individuals, the fungus triggers robust immune reactions and cause allergic rhinitis, asthma, hypersensitivity pneumonitis, and allergic bronchopulmonary

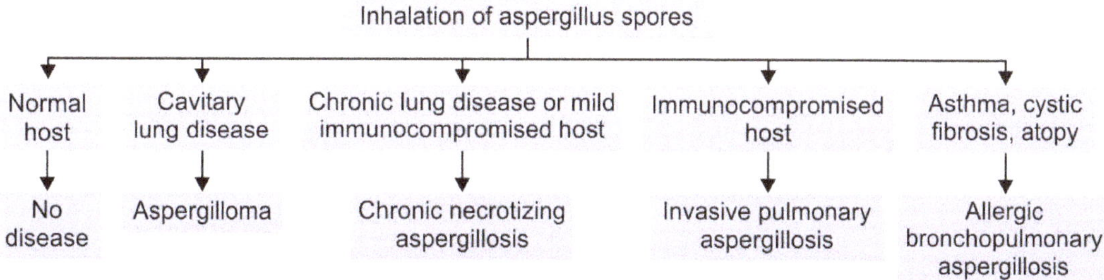

Figure 1: Spectrum of *Aspergillus*-associated lung diseases.

aspergillosis. Saprophytic growth of *Aspergillus* in pre-existing cavities gives rise to aspergilloma (fungal ball). Chronic necrotizing pulmonary aspergillosis (CNPA) occurs in patients with abnormal airways such as chronic obstructive pulmonary disease (COPD). In immunocompromised patient severe form of the disease, invasive pulmonary aspergillosis (IPA) develops. These forms represent a continuum of disease and often, there is transition from one type to the other or overlap between these forms (Figure 2).

Chronic Pulmonary Aspergillosis

Chronic pulmonary aspergillosis (CPA) manifests as chronic cavitary pulmonary aspergillosis (CCPA),[6] *Aspergillus* nodule, and simple aspergilloma. All these forms are seen in middle aged immunocompetent individuals with current or prior lung diseases. Tuberculosis and COPD are two important susceptible patient groups. Subacute invasive pulmonary aspergillosis (SAIA) is a form of rapidly progressive infection (<3 months) usually found in moderately immunocompromised patients.

Chronic Cavitary Pulmonary Aspergillosis

This clinical form previously known as complex or complicated aspergilloma was reported as a distinct entity by Denning. Chronic cavitary pulmonary aspergillosis is a form of chronic pulmonary disease characterized by new and expanding multiple cavities with or without aspergilloma. This is associated with significant pulmonary or systemic symptoms, raised inflammatory markers that lasts for at

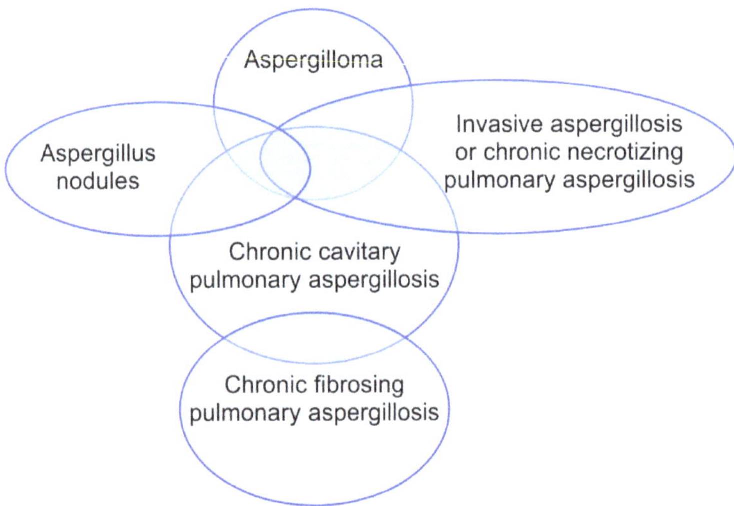

Figure 2: Clinical overlap of *Aspergillus* diseases.

least 3 months. If untreated, cavities enlarge and coalesce over years and develop pericavitary infiltrates which become fibrotic resulting in severe parenchymal destruction and pleural fibrosis. The end result of untreated CCPA is chronic fibrosing pulmonary aspergillosis (CFPA).

Radiographic findings are unilateral or bilateral areas of consolidation with multiple thick walled cavities which enlarge or coalesce with appearance or disappearance of fungal ball on serial radiology (Figures 3–5). Pleural thickening is usually seen.

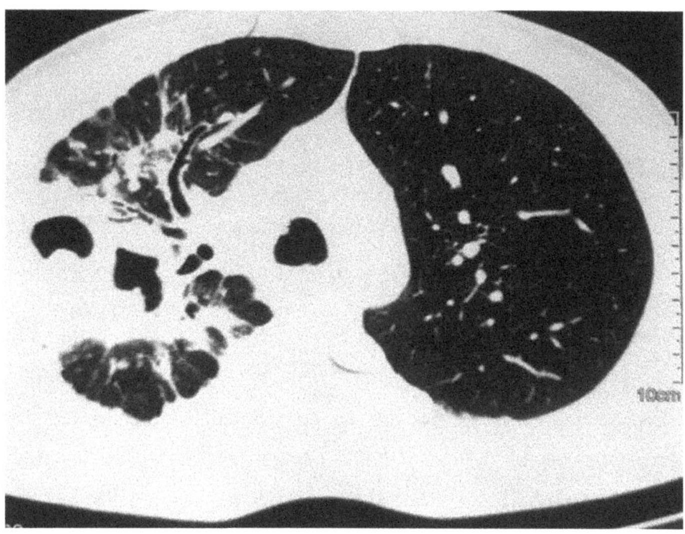

Figure 3: Areas of consolidation with cavitation and fungal ball.

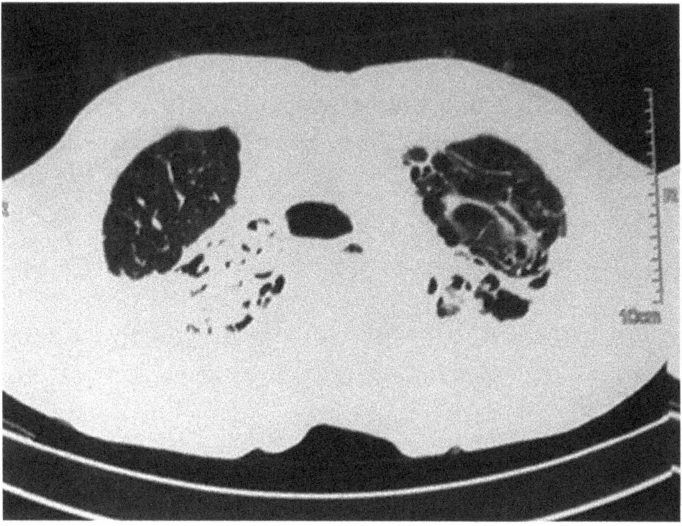

Figure 4: Bilateral upper lobe consolidation and cavitation.

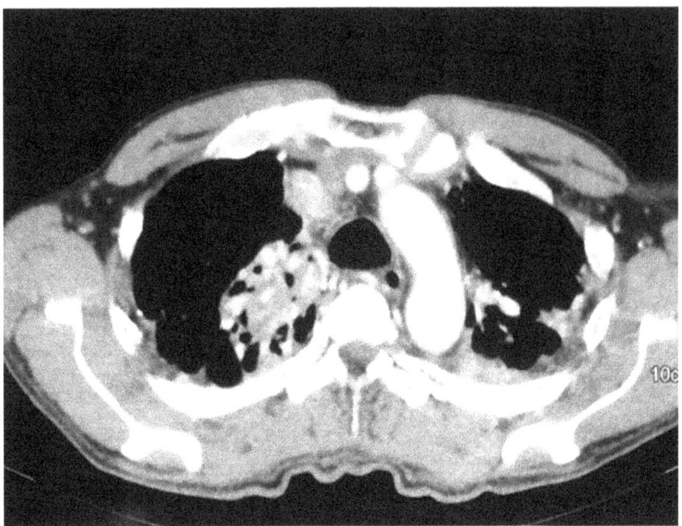

Figure 5: Upper lobe consolidation and cavitation with pleural thickening.

Chronic Fibrosing Pulmonary Aspergillosis

Chronic fibrosing pulmonary aspergillosis is usually the long term sequelae of untreated CCPA. This is classically described as extensive fibrosis of lung with destruction of parenchyma involving at least two lobes, resulting in major loss of lung function. The pre-existing cavities enlarge progressively, giving rise to large thin-walled cavities surrounded by fibrosis. The clinical course is often complicated by secondary bacterial infection or pneumothorax.

Aspergillus Nodule

Pulmonary aspergillosis can present as one or more nodules of less than 3 cm in size. Small nodules usually do not cavitate, but cavitation may be seen in larger lesions. Definitive diagnosis is by histopathology. It should be noted that sometimes rheumatoid nodules may show *Aspergillus* hyphae on histopathological examination.[6]

Chronic Necrotizing Pulmonary Aspergillosis

Chronic necrotizing pulmonary aspergillosis was previously called as semi-invasive pulmonary aspergillosis. It is an indolent cavitating infectious process which can mimic other chronic lung infections. Diagnosis is often delayed and progression to CFPA with irreversible lung damage is common. The clinical and radiological features are much similar to CCPA, but progresses much rapidly. Chronic necrotizing pulmonary aspergillosis usually occurs in mildly immunosuppressed individuals.

Predisposing conditions for CNPA:

- Diabetes mellitus
- Chronic obstructive pulmonary disease
- Advanced age
- Malnutrition
- Alcoholism
- Connective tissue disease
- Radiation therapy
- Nontuberculous mycobacterial infection
- Human immunodeficiency virus infection.

Patients present with constitutional symptoms such as fever, malaise, fatigue, weight loss, cough, and hemoptysis. Radiologically, CNPA is characterized by pulmonary consolidations, usually in the upper lobes, progressing to cavitation over weeks to months associated with bronchiectasis. Fungal ball with air crescent sign can occur due to parenchymal destruction by fungus (Figure 6).

Aspergilloma

Saprophytic aspergillosis is due to *Aspergillus* colonization of a pre-existing pulmonary cavity or ectatic bronchus. The mass is formed by conglomeration of mycelia, inflammatory cells, mucus, and cell debris. There is no tissue invasion. Patients usually remain stable or may present with intermittent hemoptysis which is sometimes massive. Chest radiography shows round or oval mass within a pulmonary cavity, with the typical air crescent sign.[7]

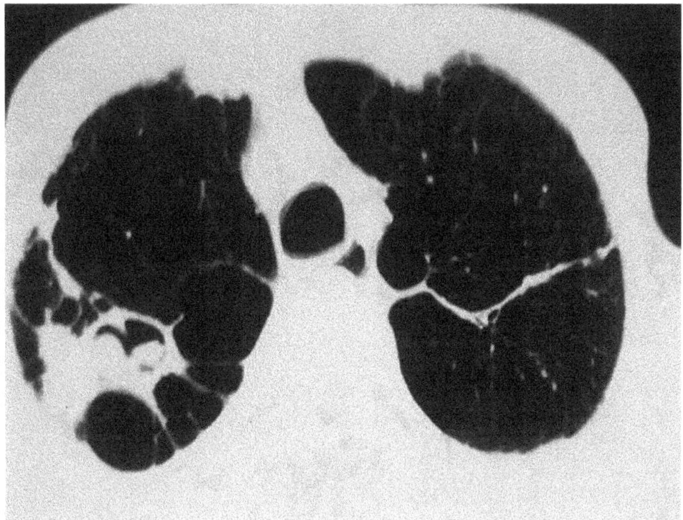

Figure 6: Upper lobe consolidation and cavitation with intralesional crescent in chronic necrotizing aspergillosis.

Invasive Pulmonary Aspergillosis

Invasive pulmonary aspergillosis is an aggressive disease due to the invasion of the bronchial wall and the accompanying vessels by the hyphae. Invasive pulmonary aspergillosis occurs primarily in patients with severe immune deficiency and is frequently seen in neutropenia and HIV infection. There is increasing number of IPA being reported among nonimmunosuppressed patients suffering from critical illnesses.

Risk factors for the development of IPA:

- Prolonged neutropenia
- Transplantation
- Prolonged and high dose corticosteroid therapy
- Hematological malignancy
- Chemotherapy
- Advanced acquired immunodeficiency syndrome
- Chronic granulomatous disease.

Invasive pulmonary aspergillosis can be either angioinvasive aspergillosis or airway invasive aspergillosis.[7] Symptoms are usually nonspecific. Prolonged fever not responding to antibiotics is the most common manifestation. Some patients develop cough, sputum, and dyspnea mimicking bronchopneumonia. Angioinvasive form can cause vascular invasion with thrombosis and small pulmonary infarcts presenting with pleuritic chest pain. Hemoptysis is an important symptom and can be mild or massive. Hematogenous dissemination to distant sites including brain may occur.

Airway invasive form accounts for 15–30% of IPA and is characterized by aspergillus tracheobronchitis (ATB) which usually occur in lung transplant patients. The three types of ATB are obstructive, pseudomembranous, and ulcerative. Pseudomembranous type is the most severe form and usually presents with cough and dyspnea. Hemoptysis is infrequent. Radiology may mimic bronchiolitis with patchy centrilobular nodules and tree in bud appearance similar to endobronchial tuberculosis. Confluence of peribronchial consolidations gives rise to bronchopneumonia like picture. Rarely, the infection is confined to tracheobronchial tree, where no radiological lesions are detectable except irregular bronchial or tracheal wall thickening. Histologically, *Aspergillus* hyphae are seen in the basal membrane.

Typical computed tomography finding in angioinvasive form is large nodules surrounded by ground glass attenuation (Halo sign) (Figure 7). Air crescent may be seen in cavitating consolidation (Figure 8). Pleural-based consolidation similar to those seen in pulmonary embolism is due to hemorrhagic infarcts. Pleural effusion is uncommon. Histologically, the lesions show invasion by fungal hyphae and vascular occlusion of small vessels by fungal hyphae.

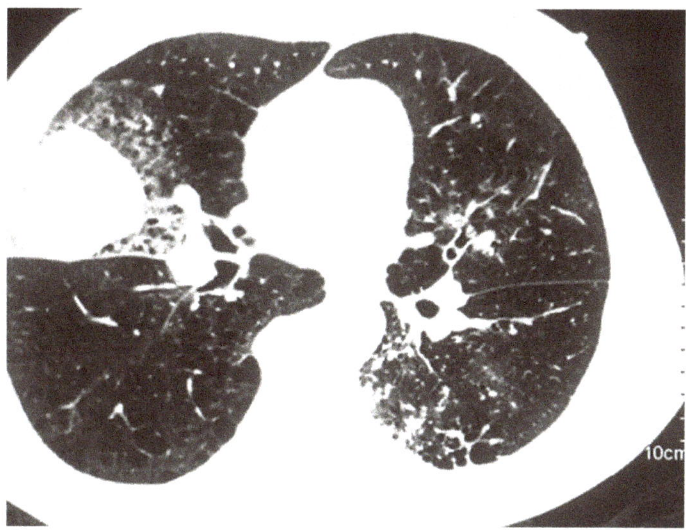

Figure 7: Angioinvasive aspergillosis with halo sign.

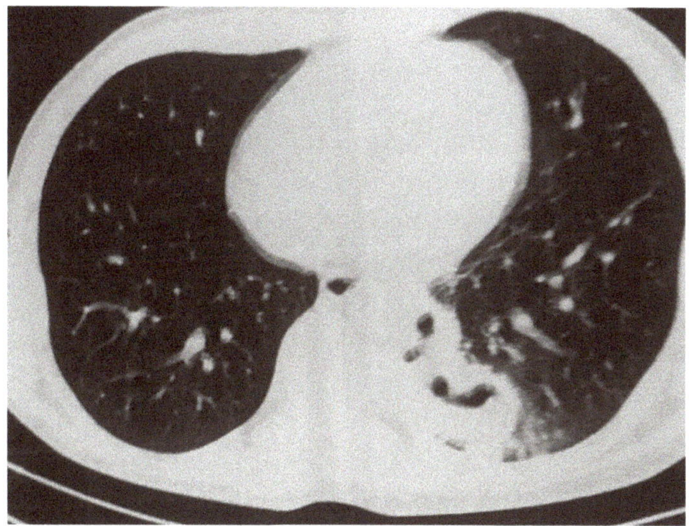

Figure 8: Consolidation with air crescent in invasive pulmonary aspergillosis.

Diagnosis

Definitive diagnosis of invasive aspergillosis or CNPA depends on the demonstration of the organism in tissue by visualization of the characteristic fungi using Gomori methenamine silver stain or calcofluor or positive culture result from sputum, needle biopsy, or bronchoalveolar lavage (BAL). In biopsy specimens, hyphal invasion of lung parenchyma confirms diagnosis of semi-invasive aspergillosis. Gold standard for the diagnosis of IPA is histopathological examination of the lung tissue demonstrating branching septate hyphae invading lung tissue. Bronchoscopic or open lung biopsy specimen may be subjected to fungal culture. Bronchoalveolar lavage fluid for fungal stain and culture is generally helpful in the diagnosis. Sensitivity and specificity of BAL fluid is 50% and 97%, respectively.

Galactomannan Antigen Test

Galactomannan testing is useful in the diagnosis of invasive aspergillosis. Galactomannan is a polysaccharide released by *Aspergillus* during growth. A positive result supports a diagnosis of invasive aspergillosis. Serum galactomannan testing is a useful test for early diagnosis and to monitor the disease during treatment. Sensitivity and specificity of galactomannan antigen assay in BAL fluid specimen is 77.2% and 77%, respectively, and in serum is 66.7% and 63.5%, respectively. The detection of (1-3)-β-D-glucan could be a promising nonculture-based, noninvasive tool for the diagnosis of invasive aspergillosis.

Treatment

The treatment of choice for simple aspergilloma is surgical resection. However, surgical resection may not be always feasible due to bilateral lung involvement, poor lung function, comorbidities, and postoperative complications.

The mainstay of treatment for CNPA and CCPA is antifungal therapy. Antifungal agents with good success rates are intravenous (IV) amphotericin, micafungin, voriconazole, itraconazole, and posaconazole. Surgery may be reserved for those not responding to medical management. In CNPA, treatment is similar to invasive fungal disease. Initial intravenous antifungal therapy should be given to treat the fungal invasion. In CCPA, oral antifungal agent is preferred. Itraconazole is ideally suited for these patients owing to the better tolerability and lesser cost. Incidence of azole resistance among *Aspergillus* strains is on the rise in several parts of the world. Azole resistance has been reported from India.[8]

The optimal duration of therapy is not yet defined. Response to antifungal therapy in CCPA is slow and a minimum of 4–6 months therapy is recommended. If there is good response, the treatment may be extended to 9 months. Studies suggest that continuing therapy beyond 6 months improves radiological response rate, but not clinical response. Relapse rate of CPA after cessation of antifungal drugs is around 50%.

In IPA, treatment should be started as soon as there is a strong clinical suspicion. First line therapy for IPA is amphotericin B. Recommended dose is 1–1.5 mg/kg/day. Amphotericin B may cause serious adverse reactions, including nephrotoxicity, hypersensitivity reactions, and electrolyte disturbances. To overcome these side effects, lipid based preparations (liposomal amphotericin B and lipid complex amphotericin B) are being used. Broad spectrum triazole, voriconazole is currently considered as the drug of choice for IPA. Prospective randomized multicenter study comparing voriconazole to amphotericin B therapy has shown better response rate with voriconazole. Voriconazole is available as oral and intravenous preparations. The recommended dose of voriconazole is 6 mg/kg twice daily intravenously on day 1, followed by 4 mg/kg intravenously till day 7. Then switch over to oral therapy at a dose of 200 mg twice daily. Voriconazole is better tolerated than amphotericin B. The most frequent adverse reactions are blurred vision and photophobia. Less frequently impairment of liver function and cutaneous reactions may occur. Drug interactions are reported with cyclosporine, warfarin, terfenadine, carbamazepine, quinidine, rifampicin, and sulfonylureas. Duration of therapy should be individualized depending on the clinical and radiological response. Prolonged treatment is often required lasting for several months to 1 year.

In refractory cases, posaconazole may be given. Echinocandins such as caspofungin, micafungin, and anidulafungin are alternate agents used if there is poor response or if the drug is not tolerated. Cases showing poor response may be put on combination drugs.

Role of surgery in IPA is limited, except with bone invasion, epidural abscess, vitreous disease or burn wounds. Other indications for surgery are massive hemoptysis, pulmonary lesions close to major vessels or heart, or presence of residual localized pulmonary lesion in candidates for immunosuppressive therapy.

Immunomodulatory therapy with granulocyte-macrophage colony stimulating factor (GM-CSF) and ϒ-interferon may be given as an adjunct to antifungal therapy. Granulocyte-macrophage colony-stimulating factor stimulate neutrophil production by bone marrow and augment the phagocytic activity of neutrophils. Another potential supportive therapy is granulocyte transfusion.

Mucormycosis

Mucormycosis is the spectrum of rapidly progressing life threatening infections caused by vasculotropic fungi of the order of mucorales. Mucorales are ubiquitous environmental fungi found in decaying organic matter. Risk factors for mucormycosis are poorly controlled diabetes mellitus, glucocorticoid therapy, iron chelation therapy, renal failure, and malnutrition.

Pathogenesis

Route of infection is by inhalation of fungal spores (3–11 μ) small enough to reach alveoli. Iron acquisition from the host is central to pathogenesis of mucormycosis.

Clinical presentation is similar to invasive aspergillosis, as pneumonia refractory to antibiotics. Massive hemoptysis due to vascular invasion is a common complication which can be fatal. Diabetics tend to present with endobronchial mass with obstruction of major airways which mimic malignancy. Diagnosis is challenging as the clinical symptoms and signs may be nonspecific. Radiological examination shows consolidation or mass like lesion (Figures 9 and 10) with reversed halo sign (central ground glass area with peripheral consolidation). Ground glass area represents lung infarction. Multiple nodules and pleural

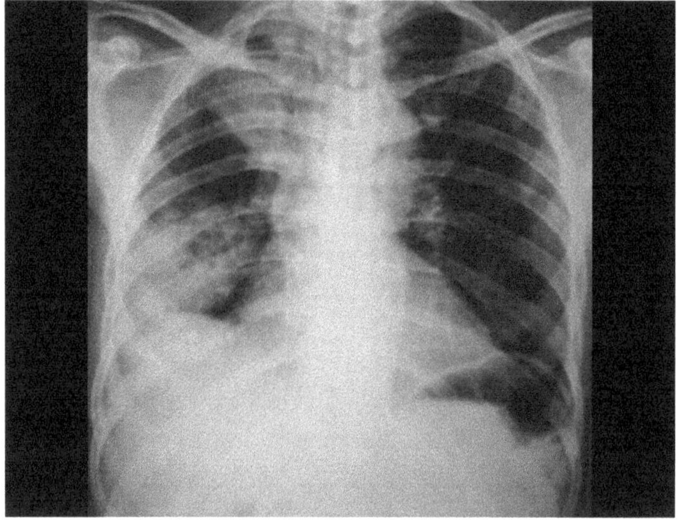

Figure 9: Showing consolidation in right upper and lower zones.

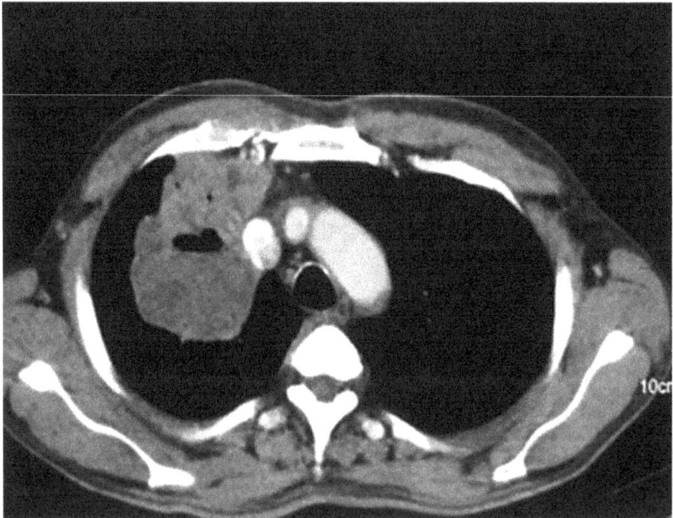

Figure 10: Computed thorax showing large mass like lesion with cavitation.

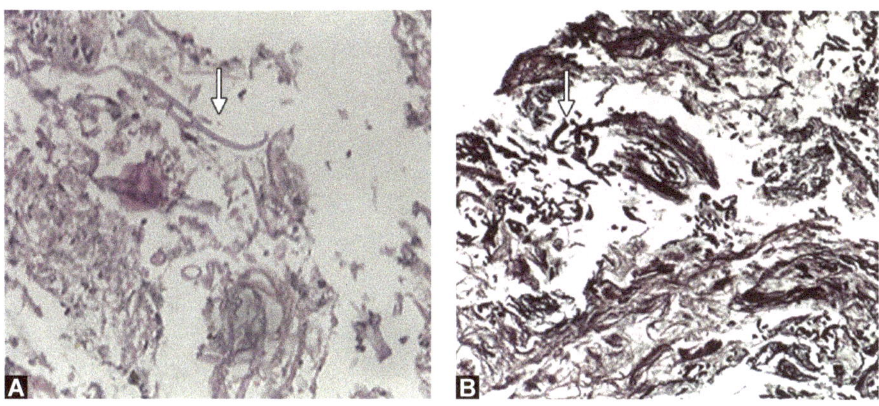

Figure 11: A, Hematoxylin and eosin stain showing mucormyces hyphae (arrow); **B,** Periodic acid-Schiff stain showing hyphae (arrow).

effusion can also occur. Serum fungal markers are negative. Definitive diagnosis is by histopathological evidence of fungal invasion by broad and nonseptate hyphae (Figure 11).

Treatment

Amphotericin B is the treatment of choice and liposomal amphotericin is given at a dose of 7.5–10 mg/kg. Posaconazole has potent activity against Mucorales. Isavuconazole is another triazole effective in management of mucormycosis, given at a dose of 200 mg three times a day for 2 days followed by 200 mg daily. Surgical debridement of infected tissue should be performed to limit spread of the lesion. Disease can be fatal even with treatment.

Candidiasis

Candidiasis is the most common opportunistic infection among immunocompromised individuals. There are over nine species of *Candida*, and *Candida albicans* is the most common species. Invasive candidiasis is a challenging problem in patients with one or more underlying diseases or surgical intervention. In intensive care unit, patients mortality rates due to *Candida* infection is reported between 20 and 40%.[6]

Pulmonary involvement of candidiasis takes the form of empyema, tracheobronchial candidiasis pneumonia and mediastinal infections.[9] *Candida* pneumonia is found in the setting of candidemia with dissemination to the lung in immunocompromised individuals. Primary *Candida* pneumonia is rare, which develops secondary to aspiration of oropharyngeal contents. Tracheobronchitis usually occurs as a complication of lung transplantation.

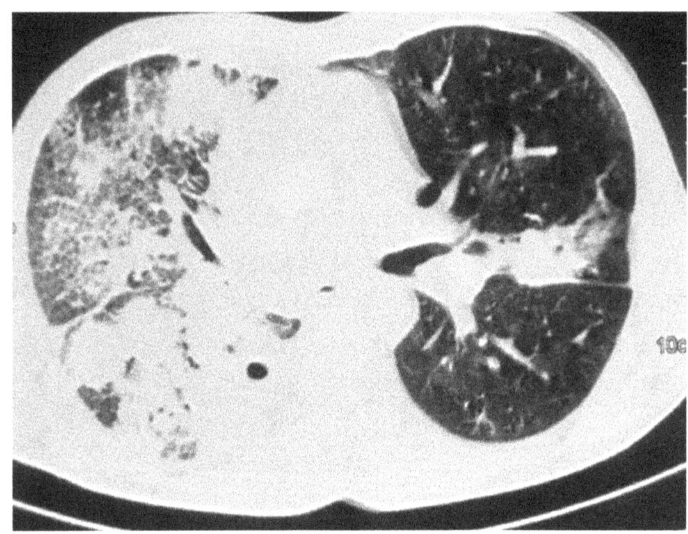

Figure 12: Showing multilobar consolidation.

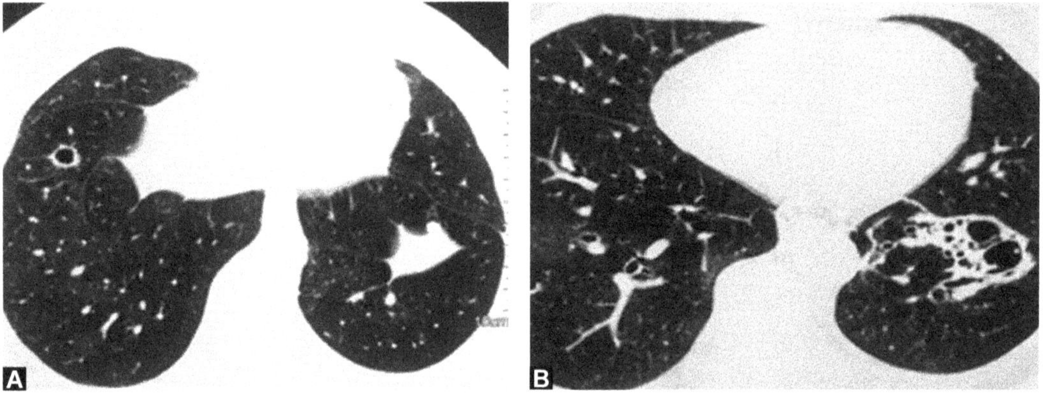

Figure 13: Pulmonary candidiasis in a diabetic female.

Clinically present with persistent fever, cough, and dyspnea. Radiographic findings are variable, showing lobar or multilobar consolidation with cavitation (Figures 12 and 13). Hematogenous spread to lungs from distant focus gives rise to random, symmetrical, bilateral nodular or miliary lesions.

Isolation of *Candida* in respiratory secretions is of limited diagnostic value, as it is interpreted as colonization. Histopathological evidence of tissue invasion is required to confirm *Candida* pneumonia. Serum β-D-glucan detection may assist to differentiate colonization from invasive *Candida* infection. However, the test has low positive predictive value, as false positivity is very high. Increasing number of infections is being reported with nonalbicans *Candida* organism such as *C. glabrata, C. tropicana, C. parapsilosis*, and *C. lusitaniae*. Some of these are inherently resistant to azole and amphotericin.

Treatment

Initial recommended treatment is echinocandin. Echinocandin loading dose is 70 mg intravenously followed by 50 mg daily for 7–14 days. Echinocandins have better safety profile than amphotericin. For candidemia, minimum duration of treatment is 14 days after the end of candidemia determined by blood culture. Removal of indwelling catheters is strongly recommended. Liposomal amphotericin and voriconazole are recommended with moderate strength for use in candidiasis.[10] Prophylactic fluconazole therapy is recommended for patients undergoing abdominal surgery and has recurrent anastomotic perforations.

Endemic Mycoses

Endemic mycoses is a group of diseases caused by diverse fungi that occupy a specific ecologic region in the environment. They exhibit dimorphism, existing as molds in the environment and as yeast or spherule at body temperature. These endemic mycoses are frequently misdiagnosed as community-acquired pneumonia[11] or sarcoidosis leading to serious consequences including mortality. Major endemic mycoses in the world are histoplasmosis, blastomycosis, cryptococcosis, and coccidioidomycosis.

Cryptococcosis

Cryptococcosis is prevalent in different parts of United States. This is caused by infection with encapsulated fungus *Cryptococcus neoformans* and *Cryptococcus gattii*. Infection is acquired by inhalation of yeast forms. Following inhalation these infective forms of the fungus reach the terminal airways, as they are smaller and less encapsulated in the environment. Fungus has worldwide distribution and grows in composted bird droppings and rotted vegetation.

Spectrum of disease ranges from asymptomatic infection in healthy individuals to diffuse pulmonary disease leading to respiratory failure and systemic dissemination in immunocompromised patients. Three forms are reported such as transient asymptomatic colonization, self-limited progressive pulmonary disease with or without systemic dissemination and cryptococcoma.

Asymptomatic cases are diagnosed incidentally when chest radiography is taken for some other purpose. Symptomatic cases, present with dry cough, chest discomfort, and low grade fever. Night sweat, hemoptysis, or weight loss may occur.

Radiologically nodular infiltrates, solid lesions mimicking pulmonary or mediastinal tumors, or abscess are most frequent. Lobar collapse due to intrabronchial mass and pancoast syndrome are two presentations mimicking carcinoma.[12] Cavitation, mediastinal adenopathy, pleural effusion, and calcification are rare.

Diagnosis is by direct demonstration of organism in biopsied or aspirated tissue. Profuse growth of organisms inside macrophages without granuloma formation is noted. Budding yeast forms with doubly refractile cell wall and clear capsule are characteristic in India ink preparation. Organism can be cultured in Sabouraud's medium. Cryptococcal antibody testing is useful and is a sensitive test. Treatment is by amphotericin B and 5-flucytosine in combination in standard doses for over 6 weeks.

Histoplasmosis

Histoplasmosis is caused by inhalation of infectious conidia or mycelia of *Histoplasma capsulatum*. Fungi grow abundantly in soil enriched with fecal matter of birds. Fungus produces two forms of yeasts, a larger one of 8–10 μ size with fine surface projections and small smooth surfaced forms of 2–6 μ in size.

Almost 75% of infections remain asymptomatic and self-limited and only 25% develop symptomatic disease. Disease manifestation is in the form of acute pulmonary disease, disseminated disease, chronic pulmonary disease, or fibrosing mediastinitis.

Acute pulmonary histoplasmosis present with acute onset fever, cough, and pleuritic chest pain mimicking acute lower respiratory infection. Symptoms usually resolve in 1–2 weeks, but in some cases persist for longer periods. In persons with impaired cellular immunity, systemic dissemination occurs resulting in weight loss, malaise, purpura, bilateral multiple nodular or fluffy infiltrates, mediastinal adenopathy, hepatosplenomegaly, anemia, leukopenia, and mucosal ulcerations. Without antifungal therapy, disease can be fatal with a mortality rate as high as 80%. A subacute form with mild symptoms which disappear spontaneously is reported in which case antifungal therapy is not warranted.[11]

Chronic pulmonary form is primarily a disease of adults with pre-existing lung disease and present with symptoms and signs similar to progressive pulmonary tuberculosis. Fibrosing mediastinitis is a benign disorder characterized by proliferation of fibrous tissue in the mediastinum. The affected patients are young adults with slowly progressive mediastinal fibrosis with invasion or entrapment of trachea, esophagus, or superior vena cava. There is associated mediastinal adenopathy. Calcification of lymphnodes is a feature in histoplasmosis.

Diagnosis

Four radiologic patterns described in chronic pulmonary histoplasmosis are infiltrative, cavitary, fibrosis with emphysema, and residual solitary nodule (histoplasmoma).

In endemic areas serology is useful. Viable organism can be demonstrated in BAL, bronchial brushings, and biopsy material. Demonstration of yeast by cytology or histopathology has high specificity but less sensitivity. Antigen testing in serum or urine is the most sensitive test in acute histoplasmosis. Antibody tests are positive in up to 90% of chronic cases.

Treatment

Most cases of acute histoplasmosis settle without treatment. Less severe infections may be treated with itraconazole or fluconazole for up to 1 year. Follow-up is needed as relapse occurs in 15% of cases.[11] In disseminated disease, amphotericin B 0.6 mg/kg daily up to a total dose of 3 g may be given.

Blastomycosis

This is caused by dimorphic fungus, *Blastomyces dermatitidis*. Although, considered endemic to Western United States, more number of cases are being reported from other parts of world including India. Natural habitat is not completely understood and it appears that fungus exists as wood saprophyte.

Clinical Features

Lung is the most common organ involved.[11] Pulmonary disease occurs most frequently in young healthy adult males, presenting as acute or chronic infection. Following inhalation of the conidial forms, symptoms start as nonspecific flu-like illness progressing to classical acute pneumonia syndrome with high fever, chills, and pleuritic chest pain. The clinical course of the pneumonia varies from self-limiting and asymptomatic to a rapidly progressive course with acute respiratory distress syndrome and shock. It may progress as chronic cavitation and necrosis mimicking tuberculosis.[11] Severe pulmonary blastomycosis is more common in diabetics and young immunocompromised patients. Chronic form lasts for weeks to months associated with fever, night sweats, chest pain, and weight loss.

Radiology

Acute form present with patchy consolidation, often bilateral, usually involving the posterior segments of lower lobes. Pleural effusion and cavitation are less frequent. Lesion may take the form of lobar pneumonia, interstitial or miliary infiltrates.

Chronic blastomycosis is associated with linear pulmonary infiltrates with dense fibrous nodular lesion or cavitary lesions and mediastinal adenopathy. Pleural involvement is common. Mass lesions with rib erosion mimicking malignancy may occur. Coin lesions and calcification are rare.

Diagnosis

Histopathological examination of biopsied material shows abscess like neutrophil collection with granulomatous response. Yeasts can be demonstrated with fungal stains.

Treatment

Acute form is self-limiting and antifungal therapy is not needed. Treatment is recommended in patients not attaining clinical resolution. In severe forms, amphotericin B is initiated and continued till clinical improvement, followed by oral itraconazole for 6–12 months.[11] However, long-term follow-up is necessary as there is chance of relapse after many years.

Coccidioidomycosis

Coccidioidomycosis is a systemic mycosis affecting human and wide range of animals, caused by *Coccidioides immitis* and *C. posadasii*. This was first reported in Argentina in 1891 in a soldier with recurrent skin tumor.[13] Disease is acquired by inhalation of aerosolized spores. After inhalation, arthroconidia transform into spherules, and these spherules on rupturing release endospore (size 2–4 μ) which can seed in any organ by lymphohematogenous spread.
There are three clinical forms:

1. Primary pulmonary
2. Progressive pulmonary
3. Disseminated.

Coccidioidomycosis mimics community-acquired pneumonia in healthy individuals and immunocompromised patients.[11] Incubation period is 10–15 days. Most common form is primary pulmonary coccidioidomycosis. Usually present as acute respiratory disease mimicking flu with cough, fever, and pleuritic chest pain (40%) or remain asymptomatic with self-limiting course (60%).[13] Lesions of primary pulmonary coccidioidomycosis generally resolve in 30–60 days without antifungal treatment. Around 50% of the asymptomatic patients develop residual pulmonary nodule. These cases are often misdiagnosed as lung cancer. Another 5% of these patients develop residual thin walled juxta pleural cavities which resolve spontaneously in 1–2 years (Figure 14). In diabetics and immunocompromised patients, the acute pulmonary form progress to chronic cavitary pneumonia. Diffuse involvement of lung also occurs by hematogenous dissemination, which can progress to respiratory failure, septic shock, acute respiratory distress syndrome, and death.

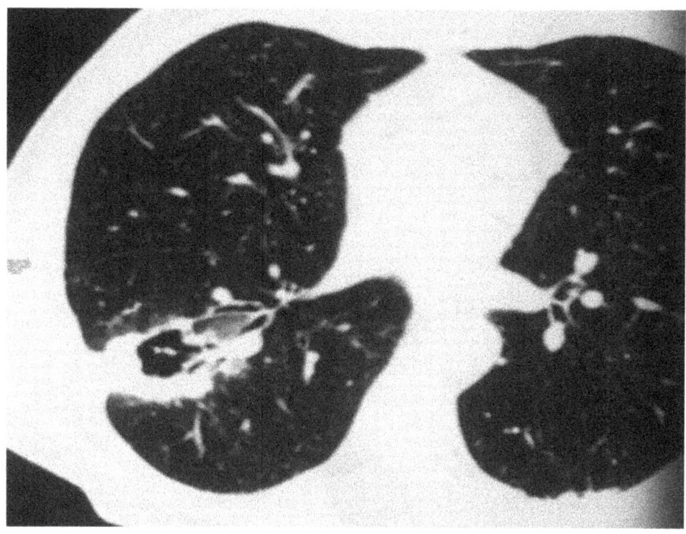

Figure 14: Thick walled cavity with adjacent ground glass area in coccidioidomycosis.

Progressive pulmonary coccidioidomycosis: Progressive pulmonary coccidioidomycosis has a chronic course and initial symptoms do not subside. Radiologically present as:

- Nodular or cavitary lesions (Figure 14)
- Cavity with fibrosis
- Miliary dissemination.

Progressive pulmonary coccidioidomycosis mimics pulmonary tuberculosis. Diabetes mellitus is a significant risk factor for this type. Other risk factors for severe disease are vasculitis, systemic lupus erthematosus, COPD, and non-Hodgkin's lymphoma.[14]

Disseminated coccidioidomycosis: In approximately 0.2% of patients with primary pulmonary coccidioidomycosis, the lesions disseminate to organs like skin, central nervous system, bones, and joints which are the most common extrapulmonary sites.[15]

Diagnosis

- Direct microscopy of sputum
- Culture due to high-risk of laboratory contamination, culture should be manipulated in class II type B2 safety cabinet. Organisms grow well in routine media

- Histopathology: Demonstration of endospores and spherules in tissues by H&E, periodic acid-Schiff and Grocott methenamine-silver (Figures 15 and 16)
- Immunological: Immunoglobulin M (IgM) precipitating antibody is positive in acute phase in 75% of cases. Compliment fixation test for Immunoglobulin G (IgG) antibody correlate with severity of lesion
- Serology for antibody is very useful for diagnosis. Immunoglobulin G or IgM antibody testing is useful.[11]

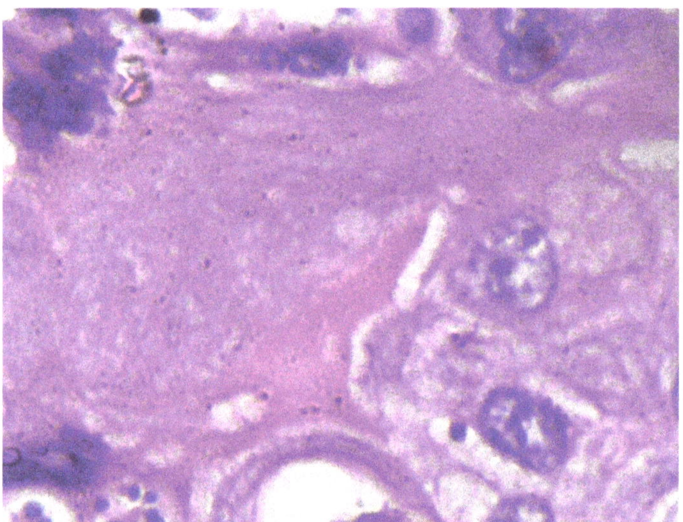

Figure 15: Coccidioidal spherules with clear halo under H&E stain (×200).

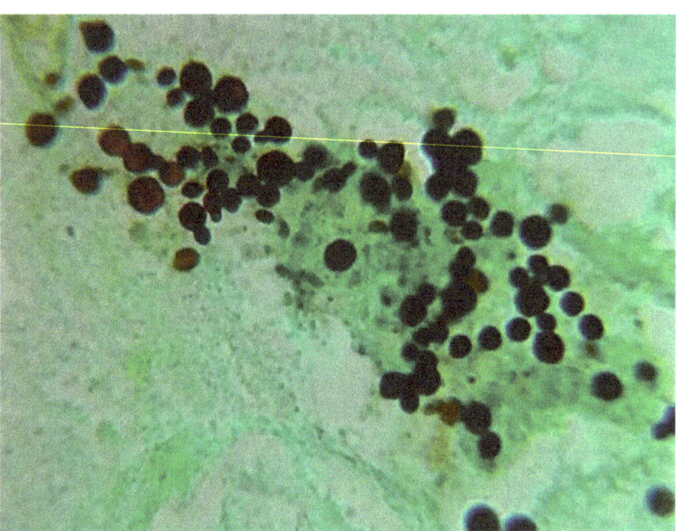

Figure 16: Coccidioidal spherules in Grocott methenamine-silver stain (magnified view ×400).

Treatment

Most patients do not require treatment other than symptomatic measures. In chronic cavitary lesions, fluconazole 400 mg/day or high doses up to 1,200 mg/day gives satisfactory results. Resection may occasionally be necessary. Itraconazole 400–600 mg/day gives slightly better results, and has lesser recurrence rates. Amphotericin B should be reserved for severe forms of the disease. Treatment should be continued for minimum 3–6 months. Long-term follow-up is recommended until completed. Prognosis is worse for diabetics and patients with cardiopulmonary disease.

Basidiobolomycosis

Basidiobolus is a fungus included in zygomycetes species and human infections due to *Basidiobolus* that are reported mostly from Africa, South America, and tropical Asia.[16] *Basidiobolus ranarum* is the pathogenic species to man. It can cause variety of clinical manifestations including subcutaneous, gastrointestinal, retroperitoneal and rarely pulmonary zygomycosis and occasionally, an acute systemic illness similar to that caused by the mucorales. No single drug was proven to be effective. Oral ketoconazole, fluconazole, or itraconazole may be of help in some cases and generally combination drugs are preferred.

ANTIFUNGAL VACCINES

There has been effort to develop novel vaccines against fungal infections. Integration of the innate and adaptive immune response of the host against fungal pathogen is calibrated and orchestrated by fine balance between the three different T cell subtypes—helper, regulatory, and effector T cells. The unique ability of the prime antigen presenting cells in the airway (dendritic cells) to initiate and orchestrate antifungal immunity of the host has positioned these cells as logical cellular targets for development of fungal vaccines.[17]

CONCLUSION

Fungal lung diseases are rapidly emerging as a new global threat. The fatal and devastating outcome of these dreadful diseases is under-recognized in the developing world due to lack of awareness and inadequate resources for research and treatment. Some respiratory diseases have possible causal association with fungal colonization such as asthma, acute exacerbation of COPD, and cystic fibrosis. The ongoing research in this field may unravel the immunopathogenesis of these so far under studied microbes and help the fight against these diseases.

Editor's Comment

Fungal pneumonias are being diagnosed with increasing frequency and is attributed to the increasing number of susceptible population as a result of widespread use of immunosuppressant drugs and devices. Organ transplant recipients and those having human immunodeficiency virus disease are also susceptible to fungal infections. Diagnosis and treatment of fungal pneumonias are often delayed as the clinical presentations are not different from other common infections. Sometimes, these infections can cause chronic pneumonia, resulting in necrosis, cavitation, and fibrosis. Pleural complications are also frequently reported. Other important concern is that opportunistic fungal organisms such as Candida species, Aspergillus species, Mucor species cause pneumonia in patients with underlying lung disease or defective host immune defenses. Newer diagnostic methods such as galactomannan and β-D-glucan, are nonculture based and should be included in the diagnostic workup of invasive fungal pneumonias. The global threat to mycotic diseases is compounded by the high cost and toxicity profile of antifungal drugs. Institution of early antifungal treatment and surgical treatment in selected cases are important in containing the infection. The author in this article reviews most of the important fungal respiratory infections highlighting the clinical and radiological picture.

Ravindran Chetambath

REFERENCES

1. Global fungal diseases. Centers for Disease Control and Prevention. National Center for Emerging and Zoonotic Infectious Diseases (NCEZID). Division of Foodborne, Waterborne, and Environmental Diseases (DFWED). Available from: www.cdc.gov/fungal/global/index.html.
2. Horn F, Heinekamp T, Kniemeyer O, et al. System biology of fungal infection. *Front Microbiol.* 2012;3:108.
3. Nguyen LD, Viscogliosi E, Delhaes L. The lung mycobiome: An emerging field of the human respiratory microbiome. *Front Microbiol.* 2015;6:89.
4. Borghi E, Morace G, Borgo F, et al. New strategic Insights into managing biofilms. *Front Microbiol.* 2015; 6:1077.
5. Wozniak KL, Olszewski M, Wormley FL. Host immune responses against pulmonary fungal pathogens. In: Amal A, editor. *Pulmonary Infection.* 2012.
6. Chronic pulmonary aspergillosis: Rationale and clinical guidelines for diagnosis and management. Task force report ESCMID/ERS guidelines 2015. Available from: https://www.escmid.org/escmid_publications/medical_guidelines/escmid_guidelines/.
7. Chabi ML, Goracci A, Roche N, et al. Pulmonary aspergillosis. *Diagn Interv Imaging.* 2015;96:435-42.
8. Agarwal R, Denning DW, Chakrabarti A. Estimation of the burden of chronic and allergic pulmonary aspergillosis in India. *PLoS One.* 9(12):e114745.
9. Shweihat Y, Perry J, Shah D. Isolated *Candida* infection of the lung. *Respir Med Case Rep.* 2015;16:18-9.
10. Cornely OA, Bassetti M, Calandra T, et al. ESCMID guideline for the diagnosis and management of *Candida* diseases in non-neutropenic adult patients. *Clin Microbiol Infect.* 2012;18S(7):19-37.

11. Hage CA, Knox KS, Wheat LJ. Endemic mycoses, overlooked causes of community acquired pneumonia. *Respir Med.* 2012;106:769-76.
12. Maziarz EK, Perfect JR. Cryptococcosis. *Infect Dis Clin North Am.* 2016;30(1):179-206.
13. Filho AD. Coccidioidomycosis. *J Bras Pneumonol.* 2009;35(9): 920-30.
14. Stockamp NW, Thompson III GR. Coccidioidomycosis. *Infect Dis Clin North Am.* 2016;30:229-46.
15. Stevens DA. Coccidioidomycosis. *N Engl J Med.* 1995;332:1077-82.
16. Chetambath R, Sarma MSD, Suraj KP, et al. Basidiobolus: An unusual cause of lung abscess. *Lung India.* 2010;127(2):89-92.
17. Roy RM, Klein BS. Dendritic cells in antifungal immunity and vaccine design. *Cell Host Microbe.* 2012;11(5): 447-56.

World Clin Pulm Crit Care Med. 2019;6(1):168-79.

Parasitic Pneumonias

[1,*] Ravindran Chetambath MD DTCD FRCP MBA, [2] Kiran V Narayan MD DM

[1] Department of Pulmonary Medicine, DM Wayanad Institute of Medical Sciences
Wayanad, Kerala, India
[2] Department of Pulmonary Medicine, Government Medical College
Kottayam, Kerala, India

ABSTRACT

Parasites, the most innocuous creatures in the natural environment, tend to cause damage to most of the major organs once they infiltrate the human body. From an isolated self-limiting eosinophilia to the most severe systemic hyperinfection and gram-negative sepsis, they always need to be an important etiological differential diagnosis in pneumonia. In this article, the authors describe the common parasitic infestations with special emphasis to lung dominant manifestations.

INTRODUCTION

Parasitic infestations of the respiratory system even though rare, are reported worldwide and are more common in the tropics. The rapid evolution of solid organ transplantation with an increasing number of immunocompromised patients, international travel, and rapid urbanization of cities has contributed to their surge. Both protozoal and helminthic infections affecting the lung can be a diagnostic challenge with varying clinical and radiologic manifestations. The migrating adult worms can cause mechanical airway obstruction, while the larvae can cause airway inflammation. A travel history to an endemic area is critical for clinicians to make a diagnosis.

ETIOLOGY

Important agents causing pneumonia are listed in table 1. However, most of the helminths and protozoa are capable of inducing lung inflammation at some stages of their life cycle

*Corresponding author
Email: crcalicut@gmail.com

Table 1: Etiological Agents for Parasitic Lung Infestation

Helminths	Protozoa
• *Echinococcus* spp.	• *Entamoeba histolytica*
• *Paragonimus westermani*	• *Plasmodium* spp.
• *Dirofilaria*	• *Trypanosoma* spp.
• *Strongyloides stercoralis*	• *Leishmania* spp.
• Schistosomiasis	• *Toxoplasma gondii*
• *Ascaris lumbricoides*	
• *Ancylostoma duodenale*	

HELMINTHIC PNEUMONIAS

Pulmonary Hydatid Disease

Human hydatid disease is caused mainly by *Echinococcus granulosus* and *Echinococcus multilocularis*. *Echinococcus granulosus* causes cystic echinococcosis mainly in liver and *Echinococcus multilocularis* causes alveolar or pulmonary echinococcosis. Humans become infected by accidentally ingesting embryonated eggs present in the feces of definitive hosts. Pulmonary/alveolar echinococcosis is caused by hematogenous spread from hepatic lesions.

Primary infection is asymptomatic and may remain as such for years, during which time lung lesions may be discovered as an incidental finding on a chest X-ray. Clinical manifestations of pulmonary hydatidosis include cough, dyspnea, chest pain, and fever. Symptoms may also occur if antigenic material is released from the cyst by either spontaneous rupture, secondary to infection or iatrogenic needle aspiration causing a hypersensitivity reaction with fever, wheeze, urticaria and rarely, anaphylaxis. Secondary infection of the cysts may lead to lung abscess or empyema. Rupture of the hydatid cysts into a bronchus may result in expectoration of cystic fluid containing parasitic membranes, hemoptysis, wheezing, respiratory distress, and persistent pneumonia.[1] Rupture of a hydatid cyst into the pleural space may result in pleural effusion, empyema, and pneumothorax.[2]

Immunodiagnostic tests using purified *Echinococcus granulosus* antigens or synthetic p176 peptide are used for diagnosis of pulmonary hydatidosis. Chest X-ray may show single or multiple cysts in the form of well-defined homogenous lesions surrounded by normal lung parenchyma (Figure 1). Posterior segments of the lower lobes are affected most frequently.[3] Classically, pulmonary hydatid cyst do not calcify, but calcification can occur over time.[4-6]

A thoracic computed tomography (CT) scan can demonstrate the ruptured cysts and daughter cysts.[7] An air crescent is formed by the collapsed laminated membranes lying detached from the pericyst (air-crescent sign). The "water

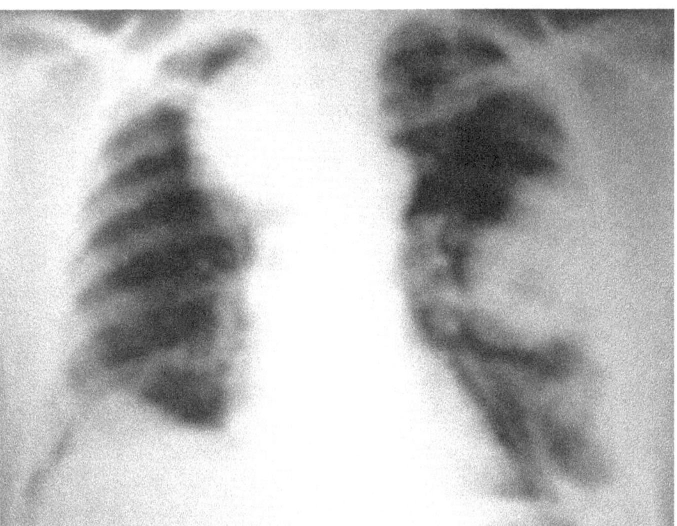

Figure 1: Multiple hydatid cysts in both lungs with left sided pleural effusion.

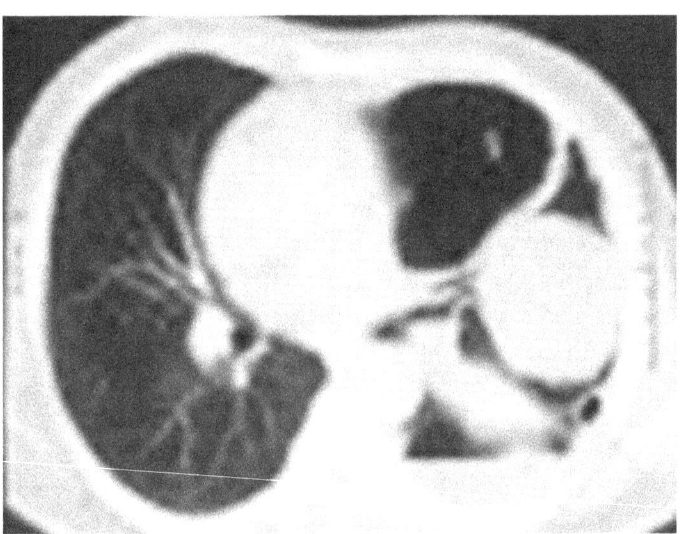

Figure 2: Computed tomography of thorax showing large cysts with pleural effusion.

lily sign" refers to the collapsed and floating laminated membranes in the cyst cavity (Figure 2). Spontaneous resolution of the hydatid cysts can occur in immunocompetent individuals, but surgical excision is preferred in most of the cases. A medical management with albendazole ± praziquantel is preferred if they are poor surgical candidates or in the presence of multiple organ involvement (Figure 3). Percutaneous aspiration followed by injection of a scolicidal agent and reaspiration (The PAIR procedure) is also successful.[8] It is also reported that

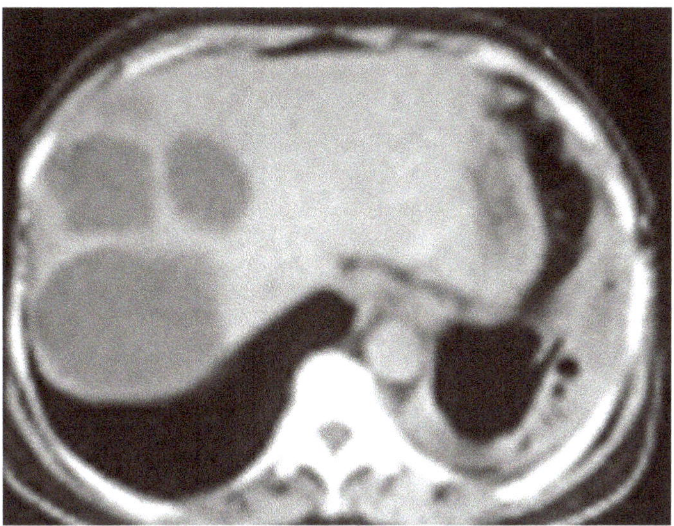

Figure 3: Computed tomography showing liver with multiple cysts.

instillation of 3% saline under thoracoscopic guidance followed by albendazole therapy is successful in pleuropulmonary hydatid disease where surgery is contraindicated.[9]

Pulmonary Paragonimiasis

Paragonimus westermani or lung fluke is endemic to Asia. Humans get infestation when they eat undercooked or raw crabs or crayfishes which are the intermediate hosts. The infective metacercariae from the human intestine passes through several organs and tissues to reach the lungs. Presenting symptoms include pleuritic chest pain, hemoptysis, chronic cough, and fever. If pulmonary cysts erode into adjacent bronchi, patients may suffer life-threatening hemoptysis (Endemic hemoptysis).[10] The chronic pulmonary form may be associated with fever, weakness, weight loss, and anemia. This clinical presentation is almost similar to pulmonary tuberculosis. Pneumothorax or pleural effusion (usually bilateral) is an important manifestation in paragonimiasis.[11]

A chest skiagram may show multifocal consolidation, cysts, ring shadows, pleural effusions, pneumothorax, and peripheral linear opacities which correspond to worm migration tracks on CT scans.[12] Low attenuation cysts filled with fluid or air in an area of consolidation can be seen on CT scans. Diagnosis is by demonstrating the parasitic eggs in stool, sputum, bronchoalveolar lavage fluid, or lung biopsy specimens. The enzyme-linked immunosorbent assay (ELISA) tests for specific immunoglobulin G (IgG) and IgM antibody are currently used for serological diagnosis of paragonimiasis.

Medical treatment is usually with praziquantel at a dose of 75 mg/kg/day for 3–5 days. Some patients may require surgery for persistent pneumothorax, pleural effusion, or empyema.

Pulmonary Dirofilariasis

Human pulmonary dirofilariasis, a disease of middle-age adults is caused by immature filarial nematodes of *Dirofilaria immitis* (dog heartworm).[2] These organisms are usually transmitted from domesticated dogs or other carnivores to humans (accidental host) by infected mosquitoes. Most patients are asymptomatic, although symptoms including chest pain, cough, hemoptysis, wheezing, fever, chills, and malaise have been reported. The most common radiological presentation is a coin lesion which is 1–3 cm in diameter and sharply defined.[13] The lesion has a central necrotic area surrounded by a granulomatous reaction and fibrous wall.[14] Dead worms may calcify. Definitive diagnosis is by wedge biopsy of tissue through video-assisted thoracoscopy or thoracotomy. Wedge resection of the pulmonary nodule is usually curative without specific medical therapy. However, some authors suggest use of ivermectin with or without diethylcarbamazine citrate for treatment.[15]

Pulmonary Strongyloidiasis

Strongyloides stercoralis is a helminth commonly found in tropical and subtropical regions and is known to cause pulmonary disease. The filariform larvae can directly penetrate through the skin, invade the tissue, penetrate into the lymphatic or venous channels, and are carried by blood stream to the heart and lungs. These larvae can pierce the pulmonary capillaries and reach the alveoli, bronchi, trachea, larynx, and epiglottis.

Infection is often asymptomatic. Respiratory symptoms may be nonspecific with wheezes and patient predominantly present with gastrointestinal symptoms.[16] In the immunocompromised patient, a systemic hyperinfection syndrome causes severe disseminated infection which may lead to gram-negative sepsis and death. These patients may develop acute respiratory distress syndrome with extensive intra-alveolar edema and hemorrhage.[17]

Radiographic findings may include miliary nodules, reticular opacities, and airspace opacities ranging from multifocal to lobar distribution (Figures 4 and 5). The definite diagnosis is made by identifying the helminth in the bronchial lavage fluid or in the stool. Antibody assays have sensitivities of approximately 90%. Patients are treated with thiabendazole, 25 mg/kg twice a day for 5 days with three courses 10 days apart followed by monthly course. Treatment with ivermectin is also effective.

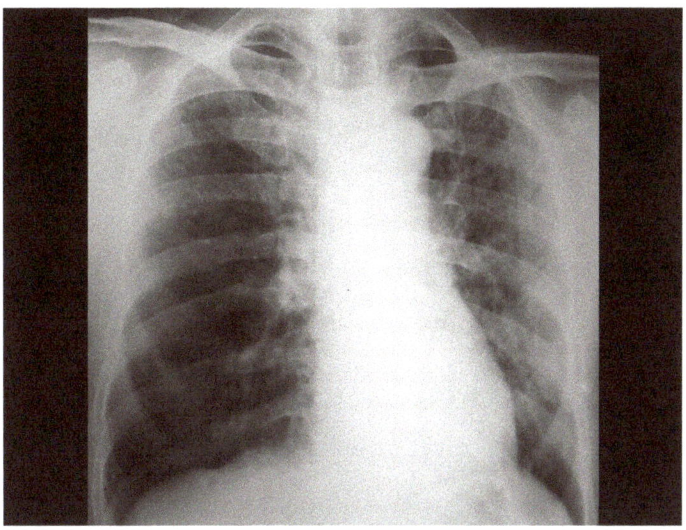

Figure 4: X-ray of an immunocompromised patient presenting with diarrhea and dyspnea. Bronchial washings demonstrated live *Strongyloides* worm.

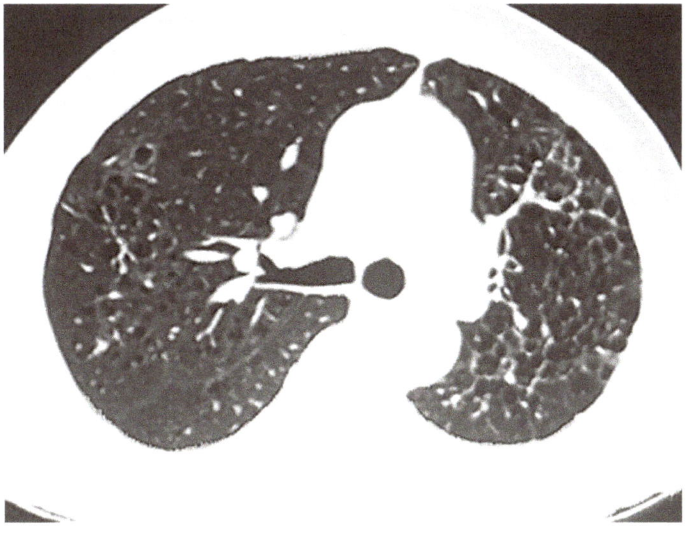

Figure 5: High-resolution computed tomography of the above patient showing small cysts and reticular shadows suggestive of pulmonary strongyloidiasis.

Pulmonary Schistosomiasis

Schistosoma species that cause human disease are *Schistosoma haematobium*, *Schistosoma japonicum*, and *Schistosoma mansoni*. Persons mostly get infected while swimming in contaminated water. Pulmonary schistosomiasis clinically presents

as an acute or chronic form. The acute form called "Katayama syndrome" or "toxemic schistosomiasis," present with dry cough, wheezing, shortness of breath, fever, chills, headache, malaise, weight loss, abdominal pain, and diarrhea. There will be radiological evidence of several small pulmonary nodules ranging from 2–15 mm in size with ground glass-opacity. The laboratory findings usually reveal 30–50% of serum eosinophilia with mild leukocytosis.
Chronic pulmonary schistosomiasis manifests in three ways:

1. Asymptomatic: Pathologically this correlates with schistosoma eggs in the pulmonary vascular tree with or without granuloma formation
2. Pulmonary hypertension: Granulomas in the pulmonary vascular bed
3. Cor pulmonale secondary to pulmonary hypertension.

The routine chest skiagram may show prominent pulmonary arteries with right atrial enlargement and a widened and elevated left heart border indicating right ventricular dilatation. Histopathology of resected pulmonary arterial specimens shows dumbbell granulomas with an interarterial and perivascular configuration. There may be local angiomatoid malformations also. Diagnosis is made by a travel history to endemic areas and a positive ELISA.[18] Diagnosis of chronic schistosomiasis is based on the identification of eggs in stool or urine by direct microscopy or by biopsy.[2]

Both acute and chronic schistosomiasis can be treated with praziquantel (20–30 mg/kg orally in two doses) and then is repeated several weeks later to eradicate the adult flukes. A short course of steroids is effective in acute form before initiating praziquantel treatment.

Pulmonary Ascariasis

Ascaris lumbricoides is the most common intestinal helminthic infestation. Infection occurs orally through the hand or food contaminated with eggs from soil. The second stage larvae penetrate the wall of the intestine and migrate to the heart and then reach lungs. The migrating larvae can induce tissue inflammation and lung granuloma formation with macrophages, neutrophils, and eosinophils.[19] This may produce hypersensitivity reaction leading to peribronchial inflammation, increased bronchial mucus production, and bronchospasm. Symptomatic pulmonary involvement may range from mild cough to Loeffler's syndrome which is a self-limiting lung inflammation associated with blood and pulmonary eosinophilia.[20]

Chest roentgenographic findings usually demonstrate basal opacities, which are bilateral, transient, or migratory. A single dose of albendazole is the treatment of choice. Mebendazole, piperazine, and pyrantel pamoate are also effective.[21]

Pulmonary Ancylostomiasis

Ancylostoma duodenale larvae can enter the human host via the oral route in addition to the skin and it can reach pulmonary circulation through the lymphatics and venules. Pulmonary manifestations are usually mild. During larval migration in the lung, the hookworm may cause symptoms and signs consistent with Loeffler's syndrome including dry cough, wheeze, dyspnea, and fever. The radiographic changes are that of Loeffler's syndrome with transient nonsegmental areas of consolidation.[14] Hookworm infestations are treated with albendazole as the first choice, a single tablet at bedtime being enough. Mebendazole and pyrantel pamoate are alternative choices.

Tropical Pulmonary Eosinophilia due to Filaria

This is a syndrome of immunological hyperresponsiveness to *Wuchereria bancrofti* or *Brugia malayi*. One of the most common causes of peripheral eosinophilia in the tropics, they are very frequent particularly in Southeast Asia.[22] Manifestations include mild fever, nocturnal cough, chest pain, rarely hemoptysis, and an absolute eosinophilia usually more than 3,000/mm^3. Tropical pulmonary eosinophilia is a differential diagnosis for miliary nodules on chest X-ray. Some previous studies of computed tomographic scan of the chest demonstrated air trapping, mediastinal lymphadenopathy, calcification, and bronchiectasis. Filarial specific IgG and IgE elevation is observed in tropical pulmonary eosinophilia. Demonstration of the live adult *Wuchereria bancrofti* in the lymphatic vessels of the spermatic cord of the patients by ultrasound examination and biopsy showing degenerating adult female worms are confirmative tests for diagnosis. The standard treatment recommended by the World Health Organization (WHO) is oral DEC (6 mg/kg/day) for 3 weeks.[23] Most patient improve with the 3 week regimen, but a sizeable proportion do not have complete resolution and may have a mild form of interstitial lung disease which can relapse also. Therefore, it is recommended to give a repeat monthly course of DEC at 3 months interval for 1–2 years.[24,25]

PROTOZOAL PNEUMONIAS

Pulmonary Amoebiasis

Entamoeba histolytica, a well-recognized pathogenic amoeba is associated with both intestinal and extraintestinal infections. Humans are infected by ingestion of mature infective cysts in fecally contaminated food, water, or hands. The cysts excyst into trophozoites in the terminal ileum and penetrate the intestinal mucosa. The most common extraintestinal manifestations of amoebiasis are liver abscess and pleuropulmonary disease. Amoebic pleuropulmonary disease can complicate approximately 15% of amoebic liver abscesses and around 1% of amoebic dysenteries. Clinical features include cough, pleurisy, shortness of breath, severe intercostal tenderness and a tender hepatomegaly.[26] The abscess is usually located in the superior part of the right lobe of liver and ruptures through the diaphragm into the right lung. This can result in a lower lobe pneumonia or a lung abscess. A hepatobronchial fistula may sometimes result in an "anchovy sauce" like phlegm.

Chest roentgenographic findings include pleural effusion, basal pulmonary infiltrates, and elevation of the hemidiaphragm mimicking a subpulmonic effusion. A combination of serological tests with identification of the parasite by polymerase chain reaction (PCR) or antigen detection is the best diagnostic approach. Metronidazole is the treatment of choice. Diloxanide furoate, a luminal amoebicidal drug can eliminate intestinal cysts. Surgical treatment of pulmonary amoebiasis may be required when there is direct pulmonary involvement or spread to pleura.

Pulmonary Malaria

The protozoa of the genus *Plasmodium* cause malaria and are primarily transmitted by the bite of an infected female anopheles mosquito to infect humans. Pulmonary manifestations of uncomplicated malaria may include subclinical impairment of alveolar ventilation, reduced gas exchange, and increased pulmonary phagocytic activity. In severe cases, there will be pulmonary edema, pleural effusion, and lobar consolidation. Complicated *Falciparum malaria* may develop acute respiratory distress syndrome. Three cases of acute respiratory distress syndrome with *Plasmodium vivax* malaria were also reported in India and one case was demonstrated with bilateral perihilar infiltrates, one case with bilateral diffuse extensive opacities, and another case with bilateral basal ground glass opacities on chest roentgenograms.[27] The alveoli are filled with parasite infested red blood cells, nonparasitic red blood cells, neutrophils, and pigment-laden macrophages. There is hyaline membrane formation in the alveoli that indicates leakage of proteinaceous fluid.[28]

Oral artemisinin-based combination therapies are the drug of choice for malaria. The WHO recommends a combination oral regimen of dihydroartemisinin with piperaquine after intravenous treatment for at least 24 hours. In addition, the WHO prefer artesunate infusion over quinine for treating severe malaria due to any Plasmodium species in all age groups.[29]

Pulmonary Leishmaniasis

Visceral leishmaniasis or "kala azar" can afflict the lung. The etiological agent is Leishmania donovani and *L. chagasi*, which are transmitted by a sand fly species

Phlebotomus. In immunodeficient hosts, it presents with nonspecific features like pneumonia, mediastinal adenopathy, or pleural effusion.[30] Pentavalent antimonials, pentamidine, amphotericin B, and miltefosine are the drugs for the treatment of visceral leishmaniasis.

Pulmonary Trypanosomiasis

Human African trypanosomiasis or sleeping sickness is caused by a protozoan called "*Trypanosoma brucei*" and "*Trypanosoma cruzi*." Pathological changes in the lung are pulmonary alveolar hemorrhage, bronchiolitis, and pneumonitis. It can cause pulmonary hypertension and dilatation of the right ventricle which is a typical characteristic of Chagas disease. Intravenous eflornithine and melarsoprol are the effective drugs for this condition.[31]

Pulmonary Toxoplasmosis

Toxoplasmosis is caused by a protozoan parasite called *Toxoplasma gondii*, which are primarily carried by cats. Humans are infected by ingestion of cyst-contaminated uncooked milk products, vegetables, or meat. The clinical manifestations are influenza-like illness, myalgia, or enlarged lymph nodes. Pulmonary involvement has been increasingly reported in immunocompromised patients. Pulmonary involvement includes interstitial pneumonia, diffuse alveolar damage, and necrotizing pneumonia. Toxoplasmosis in the first trimester results in fetal loss, neonatal chorioretinitis, and neurological problems. Diagnosis requires demonstrating the parasite in body tissues. Sputum examination can reveal the parasite in pulmonary toxoplasmosis. A real-time PCR-based assay in bronchoalveolar lavage fluid has been performed in human immunodeficiency-infected patients.[32] Toxoplasmosis can be treated with a combination regimen of pyrimethamine and sulfadiazine.

CONCLUSION

Parasitic lung diseases can mimic the clinicoradiological manifestations of many infectious and noninfectious lung diseases. Often, the only clue, a simple peripheral eosinophilia should be correlated in the correct perspective. With a multitude of extrapulmonary manifestations, they can present to various specialties like surgery, gastroenterology, hepatobiliary, skin, and ophthalmology. Touring and travel, being a hobby and leisure activity have broken the strict boundaries of regional infections. Advances in therapy and critical care have prolonged the survival of immunocompromised patients including post-organ transplants. Parasitic infections should be a consideration in this population because of the increased opportunities of infestation especially in developing nations. This article gives a brief overview of parasitic diseases affecting the lung.

Editor's Comment

The incidence of parasitic pneumonias had significantly diminished in the last few decades, but a surge has occurred in the recent times due to an increasing number of immunocompromised patients, international travel, and rapid urbanization of cities. Both protozoal and helminthic infections affecting the lung can be a diagnostic challenge with varying clinical and radiologic manifestations. Parasitic pneumonias often present with several extrapulmonary manifestations. Even though effective anti-parasitic drugs are available for most of the parasites. Pneumonias can sometimes be fatal especially when the diagnosis is delayed. It is, therefore, important to keep parasitic infections in mind especially in the developing nations and immunocompromised state.

Surinder K Jindal

REFERENCES

1. Gottstein B, Reichen J. Hydatid lung disease (echinococcosis/hydatidosis). *Clin Chest Med.* 2002;23:397-408.
2. Vijayan VK. Tropical parasitic lung diseases. *Indian J Chest Dis Allied Sci.* 2008;50(1):49-66.
3. Beggs I. The radiology of hydatid disease. *AJR Am J Roentgenol.* 1985;145:639-48.
4. Lewall DB. Hydatid disease: Biology, pathology, imaging and classification. *Clin Radiol.* 1998;53:863-74.
5. Jerray M, Benzarti M, Garrouche A, et al. Hydatid disease of the lungs. Study of 386 cases. *Am Rev Respir Dis.* 1992;146:185-9.
6. Reeder MM, Palmer PES. The radiology of tropical diseases with epidemiological, pathological and clinical correlation. Baltimore: Williams &Wilkins; 1981.
7. Erdem CZ, Erdem LO. Radiological characteristics of pulmonary hydatid disease in children: Less common radiological appearances. *Eur J Radiol.* 2003;45:123-8.
8. Mawhorter S, Temeck B, Chang R, et al. Nonsurgical therapy for pulmonary hydatid cyst disease. *Chest.* 1997;112:1432-6.
9. Lakshmanan PH, Musthafa AM, Suraj KP, et al. Pleuropulmonary hydatid disease treated with thoracoscopic instillation of hypertonic saline. *Lung India.* 2008;25(1):34-7.
10. Velez ID, Ortega JE, Velasquez LE. Paragonimiasis: A view from Columbia. *Clin Chest Med.* 2002;23:421-31.
11. Oloyede P, Inah GB, Bassey DE, et al. Comparative study of radiological findings in pulmonary tuberculosis and paragonimiasis in children in a Southern Nigeria fishing community. *West Afr J Radiol.* 2014;21:17-20.
12. Im JG, Whang HY, Kim WS, et al. Pleuropulmonary paragonimiasis: radiologic findings in 71 patients. *AJR Am J Roentgenol.* 1992;159:39-43.
13. Bielawski BC, Harrington D, Joseph E. A solitary pulmonary nodule with zoonotic implications. Chest. 2001; 119:1250-2.
14. Armstrong P, Wilson A, Dee P, et al. Imaging of diseases of the chest, 3rd ed. St. Louis: Mosby, London; 2000.

15. Johnson S, Wilkinson R, Davidson RN. Acute tropical infections and the lung. *Thorax.* 1994;49(7):714-8.
16. Lin AL, Kessimian N, Benditt JO. Restrictive pulmonary disease due to interlobular septal fibrosis associated with disseminated infection by Strongyloides stercoralis. *Am J Respir Crit Care Med.* 1995;151(1):205-9.
17. Kinjo T, Tsuhako K, Nakazato I, et al. Extensive intra-alveolar haemorrhage caused by disseminated strongyloidiasis. *Int J Parasitol.* 1998;28(2):323-30.
18. Tosswill JH, Ridley DS. An evaluation of the ELISA for schistosomiasis in a hospital population. *Trans R Soc Trop Med Hyg.* 1986;80:435-8.
19. Sarinas PS, Chitkara RK. Ascariasis and hookworm. *Semin Respir Infect.* 1997;12:130-7.
20. Ford RM. Transient pulmonary eosinophilia and asthma: A review of 20 cases occurring in 5, 702 asthma sufferers. *Am Rev Respir Dis.* 1996;93(5):797-803.
21. WHO Essential Medicines Library. 2009. Available from: http://www.who.int/medicines/publications/essentialmedicines/en/.
22. Nutman TB, Vijayan VK, Pinkston P, et al. Tropical pulmonary eosinophilia: Analysis of antifilarial antibody localized to the lung. *J Infect Dis.* 1989;160(6):1042-50.
23. Ganatra RD, Sheth UK, Lewis RA. Diethylcarbamazine (hetrazan) in tropical eosinophilia. *Indian J Med Res.* 1958;46(2):205-22.
24. Ray D. Lung functions in tropical eosinophilia. *Indian J Chest Dis.* 1974;16:368-73.
25. Vijayan VK. Tropical pulmonary eosinophilia. *Curr Opin Pulm Med.* 2007;13:428-33.
26. Mandell. Douglas and Bennett's principles and practice of infectious diseases, 7th ed. Churchill Livingstone: Elsevier; 2009.
27. Sanklecha M, Mehta N, Bagban H. Varied presentation of complicated falciparum malaria in a family. *Indian Pediatrics.* 2012;49(5):413-4.
28. Pongponratn E, Riganti M, Punpoowong B, et al. Microvascular sequestration of parasitized erythrocytes in human falciparum malaria: A pathological study. *Am J Trop Med Hyg.* 1991;44(2):168-75.
29. Kiang KM, Bryant PA, Shingadia D, et al. The treatment of imported malaria in children: *An update. Arch Dis Child Edu Pract Ed.* 2013;98(1):7-15.
30. Alvar JI, Aparicio P, Aseffa A, et al. The relationship between leishmaniasis and AIDS: The second 10 years. *Clin Microbiol Rev.* 2008;21(2):334-59.
31. Jennings FW. Future prospects for the chemotherapy of human trypanosomiasis, combination chemotherapy and African trypanosomiasis. *Trans R Soc Trop Med Hyg.* 1990;84(5):618-21.
32. Petersen E, Edvinsson B, Lundgren B, et al. Diagnosis of pulmonary infection with Toxoplasma gondii in immunocompromised HIV-positive patients by real-time PCR. *Eur J Clin Microbiol Infect Dis.* 2006;25(6):401-4.

World Clin Pulm Crit Care Med. 2019;6(1):180-97.

Aspiration Pneumonias

*Devasahayam J Christopher DNB, Shakti K Bal DNB

Department of Pulmonary Medicine, Christian Medical College and Hospital, Vellore, Tamil Nadu, India

ABSTRACT

Aspiration of oro-pharyngo-gastric contents can result in infectious complications such as pneumonia and lung abscess and noninfectious complications such as chemical, pneumonitis, bronchiolitis, and interstitial fibrosis. This article deals with recognizing the risk factors and risk-groups at play in the development of aspiration spectrum of diseases. It further describes the microbiology and management of aspiration pneumonia (AP).

INTRODUCTION

Aspiration pneumonia is an under recognized, yet an increasing problem given the demographically increasing elderly population with their accompanying comorbidities. Aspiration and its adverse effects contribute significantly to the morbidity and mortality of elderly individuals, patients with chronic respiratory disorders, head and neck malignancies, dysphagia, and neurological disorders.

DEFINITION

Aspiration pneumonia is defined as a pneumonia occurring in an individual who is at risk of aspiration or has been witnessed aspirating oropharyngeal or esophago-gastric contents into the lower respiratory tract.[1,2] "Aspiration is the event and pneumonia is the consequence."

- The event of aspiration requires two components: A compromise in the protective defenses such as cough reflex and a toxic aspirate capable of damaging the lower airways. The event of aspiration can be:

*Corresponding author
Email: djchris@cmcvellore.ac.in

Table 1: Types of Aspiration

Witnessed aspiration	Circumstantial aspiration	Suspected aspiration
History of coughing, choking after vomiting, or eating	History of vomiting, staining of pillow cover with vomitus, coughing while eating, nasogastric tube displacement	Sudden development of wheezing, breathlessness, and respiratory failure in a patient at risk of aspiration

- Witnessed aspiration, if there is history of choking after vomiting or eating
- Circumstantial or unwitnessed aspiration, if there is history of vomiting, history of nasogastric tube displacement or presence of cough while eating
- Suspected aspiration, if a person who is at risk of aspiration, but otherwise stable, suddenly develops breathlessness, wheezing, and respiratory failure (Table 1).[3,4]

SPECTRUM OF DISEASES ASSOCIATED WITH ASPIRATION

The volume and toxicity of the aspirated inoculum, the chronicity of aspiration, and the individuals' inflammatory response to the aspirated material play a role in the development of the diseases comprising the aspiration spectrum.[1] A brief description of this spectrum follows. Aspiration pneumonia is discussed separately.

Aspiration Pneumonitis

Within minutes of aspiration of acidic gastric contents (pH ≤2.5), an intense inflammatory response ensues leading to bronchoalveolar epithelial damage, alveolo-interstitial edema, peribronchiolar hemorrhage, atelectasis, and ventilation-perfusion mismatch develops.[5] The patient has sudden onset of breathlessness. Examination findings may include low grade fever, cyanosis, diffuse crepitations on auscultation, and hypoxemia. This syndrome is called aspiration pneumonitis.

Gastric acid prevents bacterial growth and hence, infection is not an issue in early stages of aspiration pneumonitis. However, extensive inflammation and lung damage lowers local defences and promotes secondary bacterial infection. A patient with aspiration pneumonitis can progress as follows:

- Rapidly worsen and and develop acute respiratory distress syndrome (ARDS) and die. It occurs in 12% of cases[6]
- Rapidly improve with clearing of the chest radiograph in 48–72 hours—occurs in 62% of cases
- Worsen after initial improvement due to secondary bacterial infection—occurs in 26% of cases. This will be seen as worsening of infiltrates on chest radiograph after initial improvement.

Management is by clearing the upper airways to remove particulate matter and fluids, endotracheal intubation in patients who are unable to protect their airways, supportive care with oxygen, nebulizations, and chest physiotherapy.[1] It is difficult to differentiate aspiration pneumonitis from AP based on symptoms[3] and thus, the physician has to take a difficult decision on giving antibiotics and corticosteroids.

Antibiotics are not required in the management of early aspiration pneumonitis as the gastric acid makes the aspirated inoculum sterile. One-fourth of the patients with aspiration pneumonitis develops secondary bacterial infection and worsen after initial clinical improvement. Considering all these factors, the following decision rule can help in deciding antibiotics:

- Start antibiotics after an event of witnessed or suspected aspiration, especially if the patient is severely ill
- If no radiological infiltrates develop after 48–72 hours, antibiotics can be discontinued
- If a radiological infiltrate was initially present but the clinical condition rapidly improves, then repeat chest X-ray should be done to document radiological improvement and antibiotics can then be discontinued.

Continuing antibiotics in cases of aspiration pneumonitis does not improve outcomes and may expose the patient to harm antimicrobial therapy.[7]

The role of corticosteroids in aspiration pneumonitis is debatable. In cases of "pure" aspiration pneumonitis without any bacterial superinfection, such as seen in vomiting after drug over dosage, steroids may help early resolution of respiratory failure.[1,8] However, if a patient who is premorbidly dysphagic with poor oral hygiene develops aspiration, infectious complications are more likely and corticosteroids will worsen the outcomes.[8] Low dose steroids can be given if the patient develops ARDS.[1]

Mechanical Obstruction

Fluid and solid matter in the aspirated inoculum may lead to mechanical obstruction or reflex vagal mediated airway obstruction leading to transient hypoxemia. This sudden obstruction may occasionally trigger pulmonary edema further worsening the respiratory failure. Treatment of this condition is supportive with 100% oxygen, positive pressure ventilation, and isoproterenol to abolish the vagal reflex. Mechanical obstruction by solid particulate matter leading collapse of segments or lobes will necessitate bronchoscopic removal or the foreign bodies to relive the obstruction.

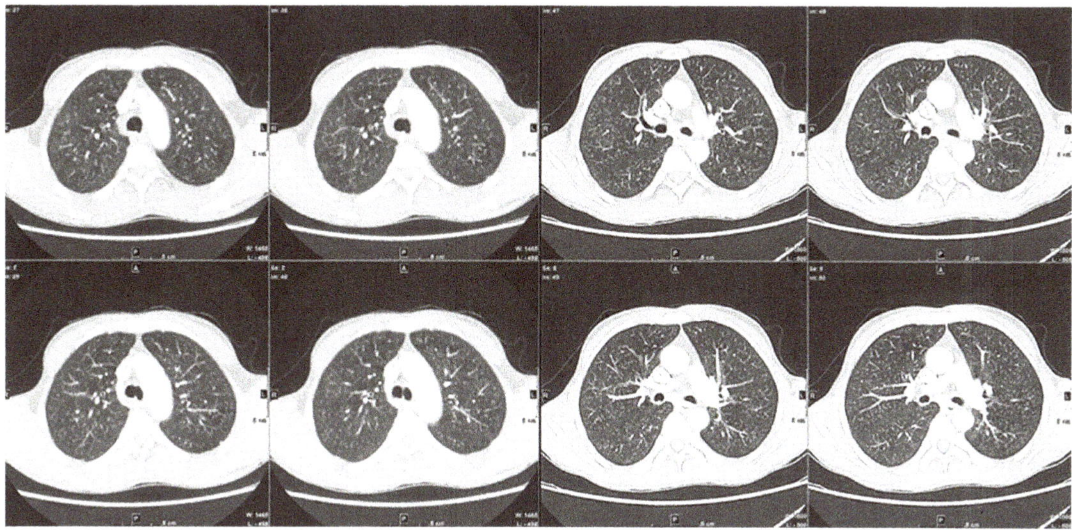

Figure 1: A 43-year-old man with carcinoma hypopharynx with cough. Routine computed tomography revealing features of diffuse aspiration bronchiolitis in all lobes.

Diffuse Aspiration Bronchiolitis

Chronic occult aspiration can sometimes result in bronchiolar inflammation and this manifests as episodic breathlessness, cough with expectoration and bronchospasm in patients (usually elderly) who are predisposed to aspiration[1,9] such as those having neuro-esophageal disorders leading to swallowing impairment, psychotropic drug abuse, gastroesophageal reflux disease, etc. High resolution computed tomography (CT) thorax will show bronchiolar thickening, centrilobular nodules, and tree-in-bud opacities predominantly in the lower lobes (Figure 1). Occasionally, diffuse distribution or upper lobe distribution of these nodules can be seen.[10] Obstructive pattern in flow-volume loop is common and may have associated reduced diffusion capacity for carbon monoxide.

Interstitial Fibrosis

Chronic occult aspiration followed by inflammation and fibrosis can frequently result in interstitial fibrosis, the pattern of which can be described as a usual interstitial pneumonia, nonspecific interstitial pneumonia, or unclassifiable interstitial fibrosis.[10]

Organizing Pneumonia

Peripheral patchy lower lobe predominant areas of consolidation in a broncho-vascular distribution can occur in patients with chronic aspiration.[11] More often, organizing pneumonia is an accompanying feature with other diseases of the aspiration spectrum.[10]

Diffuse Pulmonary Ossification

Chronic aspiration, inflammation, and fibrosis may lead to the formation of calcified nodules in a tree-in-bud pattern (nodules along the bronchovascular nodules) or nodular pattern (nodules in alveolar spaces).[11,12] This is called diffuse pulmonary ossification.

Exogenous Lipoid Pneumonia

The free fatty acids in the aspirated inoculum trigger an inflammatory process and depending upon the volume and chronicity of the oily aspirates, this can present as an acute pneumonia (large aspirate), ground-glass opacities with interlobular septal thickening crazy-paving appearance, mass-like opacities, or consolidation with fat attenuation (<10 Hounsfield units) in CT thorax.[11] This condition can occur in individuals who use laxatives and nasal drops with an oil base, fire-eaters, occupational settings that involve spraying of pesticides or paints or in those who are predisposed to aspiration due to anatomic or functional defect in swallowing.[13]

ASPIRATION PNEUMONIA

Aspiration pneumonia denotes an infectious complication as opposed to noninfectious consequence such as aspiration pneumonitis. The following section details out the risk factors, risk groups, microbiology, and management of AP.

Risk Groups and Risk Factors Responsible for Aspiration Pneumonia

Two central pillars in the development of AP are oropharyngeal dysphagia and oropharyngeal colonization by pathogenic microbiota (Table 2).[14] All risk factors end up causing one or the other. An outline of the risk groups and risk factors for AP are given in table 2.

Aspiration Pneumonia in Elderly

Aspiration pneumonia in the elderly is closely related to their level of functional decline.[15] The following factors are associated with increased risk of AP in elderly:[16]

- Increasing age and male sex

Table 2: Risk Factors for Aspiration Pneumonia

Suspect aspiration pneumonia when pneumonia develops in the background of a swallowing disorder and oropharyngeal colonization.

Suspect swallowing disorder when:	Suspect oropharyngeal colonization when:
• Esophageal disorders	• Poor oral hygiene
• Stroke	• Oropharyngeal candidiasis
• Dementia	• Dry mouth
• Altered consciousness	• Nasogastric tube feeding
• Movement disorders	• Malnutrition
• Psychotropic medications	• Usage of inhaled anticholinergics and inhaled steroids
• Head and Neck malignancies	• Ventilated patients
• Severe chronic lung diseases	

- Lung diseases: Severe chronic obstructive pulmonary disease (COPD) is associated with impaired coordination between inhalation and deglutition. Anticholinergics lead to xerostomia, increased bacterial colonization, and swallowing dysfunction
- Dysphagia: Dysphagic elderly are 12 times more likely to develop AP.[17] Dysphagia can be caused by neurological diseases, oro-pharyngo-esophageal malignancies, and antipsychotic drugs. Dysphagia leads on to a vicious cycle of malnutrition which leads to further muscle weakness, dysphagia, and AP15
- Neurological illnesses: Parkinson's disease, dementia, and stroke all predispose to increased incidence of AP
- Malnutrition: Increased chance of associated infections and reduced respiratory muscle strength can occur with protein-energy malnutrition, thus increasing the chance of AP
- Diabetes mellitus
- Proton pump inhibitor usage is associated with increased gastric microbial colonization and increased chance of AP
- Poor dental hygiene: Decayed teeth, gingivitis, plaques, and poorly maintained dentures leads to colonization with aerobic and anaerobic pathogens[17] and increased risk of AP.[16]

Aspiration Pneumonia in Head and Neck Cancer Patients

In contrast to neurological disorders, where aspiration occurs before or during swallowing, aspiration in head and neck cancer (HNC) patients occurs after swallowing. During this phase, excess residual material of the food bolus, which has not passed into the esophagus, passes into the larynx above the vocal cords or below the vocal cords. Oropharyngeal dysphagia in such patients leads to malnutrition, dehydration, poor dental hygiene, and these again promote AP.[18]

Factors that predispose AP in patients with head and neck malignancies include:

- Patient related factors: Alcoholism, smoking, poor dental hygiene, pretreatment hypoalbuminemia, usage of sleeping pills, and presence of coexisting other organ malignancies[19]
- Malignancy related factors: Cancer of the tongue, buccal mucosa, oropharynx and larynx, the T and N staging[18,20]
- Treatment related factors: Can be cancer-specific treatment related and supportive-treatment related
    - Cancer-specific treatment related predisposing factors include:
        - Surgical factors: Surgery of base of the tongue, resection of arytenoids, cranial nerve disruption will worsen oropharyngeal dysphagia
        - Chemoradiotherapy (CRT) of HNC leads to oral mucositis, sub-mucosal edema and mucosal fibrosis, dysfunction of the tongue, pharyngeal, and laryngeal muscles thus, worsening swallowing dysfunction.[20,21]
    - Supportive treatment related factors: Nasogastric tube feeding; drugs such as anticholinergics and inhaled steroids promote xerostomia and hence, poor oral hygiene and dysphagia; and antidepressants and sedatives which depress sensorium.

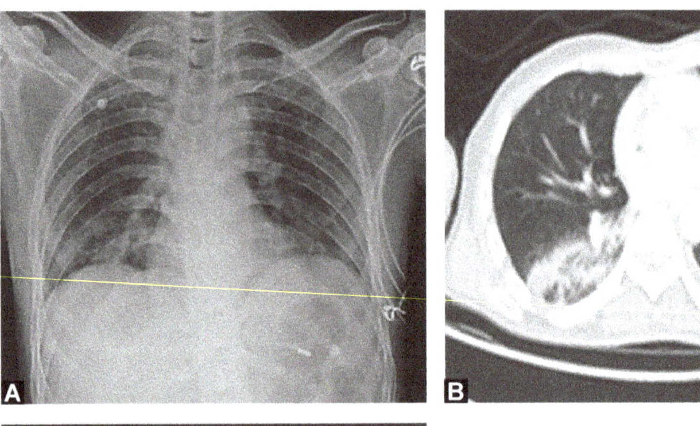

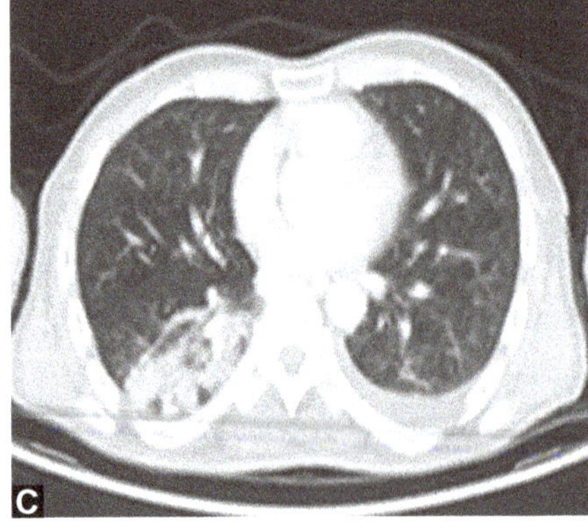

Figure 2: Patient admitted with inflammatory myopathy with bulbar involvement leading to dysphagia to solids and liquids. **A,** Chest X-ray; **B** and **C,** Computed tomography of thorax revealed pneumonia in the superior segment of right lower lobe.

Aspiration Pneumonia in Patients with Neurological Disorders

Aspiration pneumonia can occur in any neurological illness associated with altered sensorium or swallowing dysfunction (Figure 2). It has been best studied in the context of stroke (ischemic and hemorrhagic), Parkinson's disease, and cerebral palsy.

- Post-stroke AP: Available evidence suggests that pneumonia in the stroke setting is predominantly AP.[22,23] The incidence of pneumonia in the first week after stroke is around 10%.[24,25] Around 50% of the stroke patients have dysphagia of whom 50% develop AP. However, 50% of those who develop AP following stroke do not have dysphagia.[24] Nasogastric tube (with or without feeding), nil by mouth status, stroke induced immunosuppression are additional contributors[23]
- Parkinson's disease: Aspiration pneumonia accounts for 70% of deaths occurring in patients with Parkinson's disease. These patients have swallowing difficulties, weakened cough due to rigidity of chest wall, dysfunction of masticatory muscles leading to pooling of saliva, drooling and aspiration, and impaired coordination between inhalation and deglutition leading to swallowing during inhalation[26]
- Cerebral palsy (CP): A 40–70% of the patients with cerebral palsy develop AP.[27] Impairment of oral movements, pharyngeal phase of swallowing, ventilatory coordination of swallowing are all found in patients with CP. Chronic aspiration and its associated consequences such as chronic cough, impaired sleep, diffuse aspiration bronchiolitis, and pseudomonas colonization of the respiratory tract and progressive parenchymal damage can be seen in such patients.[27,28]

Aspiration Pneumonia in Ventilated Patients

Ventilator-associated pneumonia (VAP) is basically AP where micro-aspiration or silent aspiration of these bacteria laden secretions through the space between the endotracheal tube and trachea lead to the development of pneumonia.[29] Pathogenic microbiota colonizing the oropharynx, dental plaques, sinuses (due to presence of nasogastric tube) and the stomach (due to the usage of peptic ulcer prophylactic measures), high gastric volumes, underinflated cuff, supine positioning, and poor oral hygiene increase the risk of VAP.

Microbiology of Aspiration Pneumonia

Elderly

Majority of the pathogens in AP are gram-negative pathogens such as *Haemophilus influenzae*, *Klebsiella*, *Escherichia coli*, and *Enterobacter* with a lesser

Table 3: Approach to Management of Aspiration Pneumonia
Send appropriate (sputum or BAL fluid) microbiological samples
• Check for risk factors for multidrug resistance pathogens
• Check for tuberculosis
• Attempt to differentiate from aspiration pneumonitis
Remember: Role of gram-negatives > gram positive > anaerobic organisms in aspiration pneumonia.

role of anaerobes (Table 3). In a study of institutionalized elderly patients with similarly distributed moderately poor levels of oral hygeine, El-Solh et al.[30] found that gram-negative enteric bacilli were the predominant organism in 49% of cases and anaerobic organisms were predominantly found in 16% of cases. Fifty-five percent of the anaerobic isolates had concurrent growth of gram-negative bacteria. Regimens without anaerobic cover were not associated with poorer outcomes if gram negative cover was instituted. Implicated anaerobic organisms include *Prevotella, Fusobacterium, Peptostreptococcus*, and *Bacteroides*.[31]

Multidrug resistant pathogens are implicated in AP in patients with the following risk factors:[32]

- Antibiotics within the previous 90 days
- Currently hospitalized for 5 or more days
- High-frequency of antibiotic resistance in hospital
- Hospitalized 2 or more days within the previous 90 days
- Residence in nursing home
- Home infusion therapy
- Chronic dialysis
- Home wound care
- Family member with multidrug resistant (MDR) pathogens
- Immunosuppressive disease or therapy.

Clinical Features

After an event of aspiration, an attempt must be made to distinguish AP from aspiration pneumonitis as both can present with cough, breathlessness, wheezing, and oxygen desaturation. Diagnostic dilemma arises because of fewer or more indolent symptoms, symptoms of comorbidities such as congestive cardiac failure or COPD. New onset tachypnea, hypoxemia, fever, change in mental status unexplained by other causes, loss of appetite, and lethargy should alert one to the possibility of an AP.[3,33] Pleuritic chest pain is uncommon in this population.[34] Anaerobic infections should be suspected when there are indolent symptoms, absence of rigors, putrid sputum with negative growth on cultures, poor oral hygiene, and radiological evidence of abscess and empyema. Rapid progression of symptoms may suggest infection with *Staphylococcus aureus* and *Psueodomonas*. However, one should not attempt to tailor the antibiotics based on the symptoms and signs, alone. El-Solh et al.[30] found similar degrees of hypoxemia, severity of illness, distribution, and rates of worsening of radiological opacities in patients with AP due to gram negative infections or anaerobic infections.

Diagnosis

There is no specific test to diagnose AP, and for diagnosis a combination of clinic-radiological-microbiological tests should be taken together with demonstration of oropharyngeal dysphagia.

Blood Tests

Elevated total leukocyte counts, serum procalcitonin, and C-reactive protein (CRP) along with decreased serum albumin levels can be seen. Serum procalcitonin is elevated both in aspiration pneumonitis (due to the intense inflammatory reaction induced by the gastric acid) and AP (bacteria mediated inflammation related) and hence, cannot be used to differentiate one from the other.[35] However, serum procalcitonin levels fall in parallel with the rapid resolution of aspiration pneumonitis. A persistently elevated serum procalcitonin after 72 hours of onset of pneumonia/pneumonitis indicates superadded or primary bacterial infection.[35]

Radiology

According to a recent study on 53 patients,[36] AP presented as:

- Bronchopneumonia (peripheral and peribronchiolar air space consolidation of one or more segments of one or more lobes)—68% of cases
- Centrilobular nodules with tree-in-bud appearance—17% of cases
- Lobar pneumonia—15% of cases.

Aspiration in an upright or semirecumbent position that will affect the basal segment of the lower lobes. Diffuse distribution of opacities can be seen in patients with latter being found in patients with poor performance status. Aspiration in a supine position will affect the posterior segments of the upper lobes and superior segment of the lower lobes (Figures 3 and 4).[11] Anterior and upper lobe distribution is not consistent with AP.

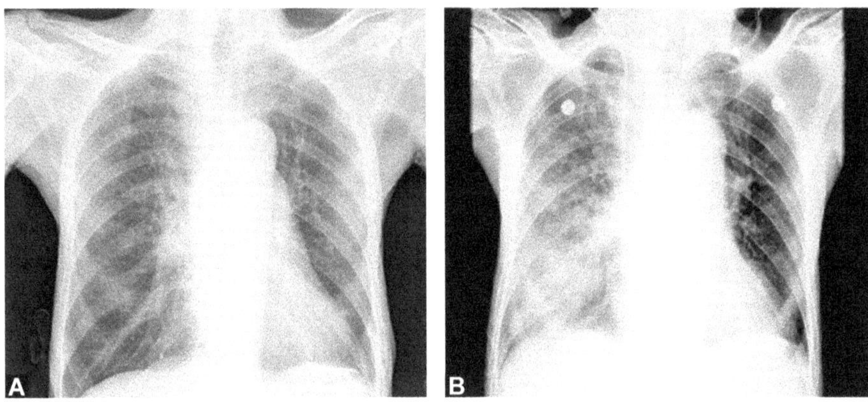

Figure 3: A 60-year-old severe chronic obstructive pulmonary disease patient with: **A,** Type II respiratory failure at admission improving on biphasic positive airway pressure developed vomiting and aspiration pneumonia, and sudden worsening of respiratory failure; **B,** Chest X-ray showing right lower lobe consolidation.

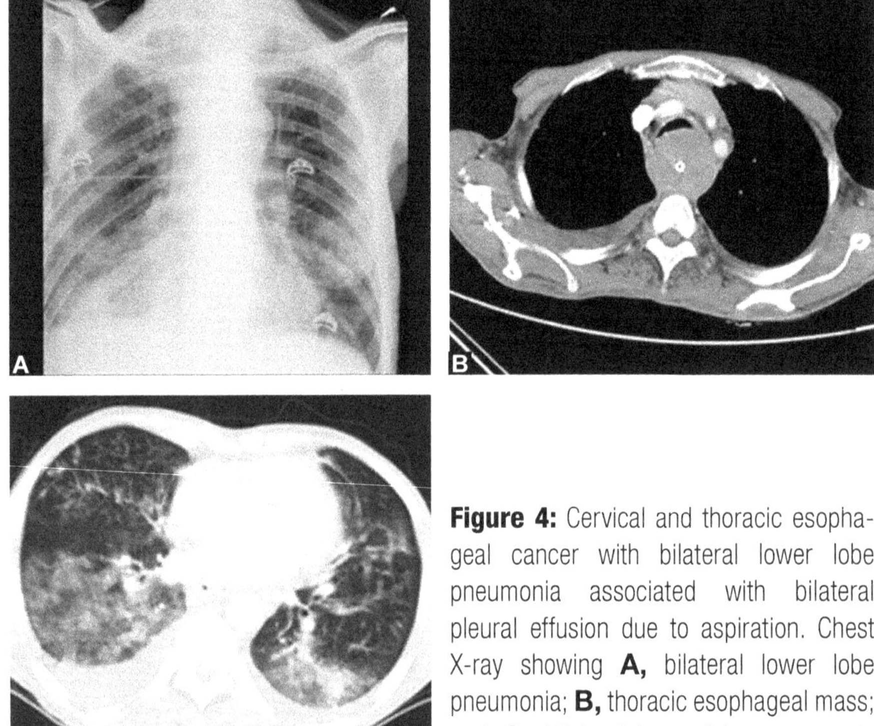

Figure 4: Cervical and thoracic esophageal cancer with bilateral lower lobe pneumonia associated with bilateral pleural effusion due to aspiration. Chest X-ray showing **A,** bilateral lower lobe pneumonia; **B,** thoracic esophageal mass; and **C,** bilateral lower lobe pneumonia with bilateral pleural effusion.

Microbiology

Microbiological samples can be obtained by sputum culture, fiber optic bronchoscopy guided bronchoalveolar lavage, or pleural fluid cultures in cases of empyema. Tuberculosis must be ruled out. Anaerobic cultures are logistically difficult and not done routinely.

Dysphagia or Swallowing Disorder Screening

The need for evaluating a swallowing disorder can be seen in the following scenarios:

- Diagnostic evaluation of a disease belonging to the aspiration spectrum, e.g., in identification of the cause of unexplained bronchiolitis in an elderly patient
- Planning management, e.g., deciding when to resume oral feeds after a cerebrovascular event.

The evaluation of a swallowing disorder (Table 4) is best done by a speech language pathologist. A brief outline is given in table 4.

Bedside Assessment

- Before proceeding to specific bedside tests, the clinician should, if possible, observe the patient during a meal. Prolonged meal times, incomplete meals, difficulty in chewing and multiple swallows per bite, nasal regurgitation, coughing (immediate or delayed) or choking during eating, and voice changes post swallowing can be suggestive of a swallowing disorder.[37] The clinician can then perform a brief examination of those cranial nerves associated with swallowing—V, VII, IX, X, XI, and XII nerves
- Specific beside tests: Water swallow tests can be performed at the bedside with end points of coughing, choking, voice change or desaturation post swallowing as indicative of aspiration.[37,38] Single sips of small volumes (1–5 mL) or larger volumes (5–20 mL), multiple interrupted sips tests of larger volumes (50 mL), or tests of uninterrupted consecutive sips of large volumes (90–100 mL) can be performed. The presence of clinical signs of aspiration on drinking small single sips confirms aspiration. The absence of clinical signs of aspiration after uninterrupted swallowing of large volumes rules out aspiration.[37]

Table 4: Screening for Swallowing Disorders

Bedside assessment	Specific imaging tests
• Observe the patient during a meal for red flag signs or symptoms • Cranial nerve examination—V, VII, IX, X, XI, XII • Water swallowing tests: Single sips of small volumes (1–5 mL or 5–20 mL), multiple interrupted sips amounting to larger volumes (50 mL), or uninterrupted sips of large volumes	• Functional endoscopic sinus surgery • Videofluoroscopic swallowing

Specific Imaging Tests

Two tests deserve mention—modified barium study (MBS, also known as the videofluroscopic of swallowing study or VFS) and the fibreoptic examination of swallowing (FESS). Barium coated foods are swallowed during MBS and colored foods of various consistencies can be used during FESS. These tests allow the clinician to directly observe the swallowing process and quantitate aspiration by means of quantifying the penetration (food residue in the laryngeal vestibule) and aspiration (food residue below the vocal cords).[39]

Treatment and Prevention of Aspiration Pneumonia

The following section is divided into antibiotic therapy and other supportive and preventive pharmacologic and nonpharmacologic measures.

Antibiotic Therapy

The most common causative organisms in AP are the gram-negative bacteria followed by gram-positive bacteria. The role of anaerobic bacteria is being seen more as colonizing oropharyngeal flora or as coinfection. However, anaerobic coverage is clearly indicated in classic aspiration pleuropulmonary syndromes especially when there is a history of loss of consciousness in patients with coexisting gingival disease or esophageal motility disorders.[40]

Three principles need to be remembered (Table 5):

- Single or universal anaerobic agent cover is not advisable
- Fluoroquinolones should not be given until tuberculosis has been appropriately ruled out
- Aerobic gram negatives should be covered as they are the most common organisms found to be causative.

Hence, the first choice antibiotics include ampicillin-sulbactam (1.5–3 grams every 6 hours for those with normal renal parameters) followed by coamoxi-clavulanate (1 gram twice daily) after oral intake is not contraindicated. If the patient is allergic to penicillin then clindamycin (600 mg intravenous every 8 hours) can be given. For those with nosocomial pneumonia or with risk factors for multidrug resistant pathogens (see above), a carbapenem (meropenem) or piperacillin-tazobactam may be used. All these agents have the additional benefit of covering all the respiratory anaerobic infections.

Agents with anaerobic coverage increase the risk of *Clostridium difficile* infection and it is prudent to limit its use to the required duration. The ideal duration of antibiotic treatment without the necrotizing pleuropulmonary

Table 5: Treatment and Prevention of Aspiration Pneumonia

Treatment

- Three principles
  - Universal anaerobic cover or single limited anaerobic cover should not be used
  - Fluroquinolones should not be used until tuberculosis has been conclusively ruled out
  - Aerobic gram-negative coverage should be given as the first-choice agent
- First choice agent
  - No risk factors for multidrug resistant (MDR) pathogens: Ampicillin-clavulanate/ clindamycin (if penicillin allergy)
  - Risk factors for MDR pathogens: Meropenem or piperacillin-tazobactam
- Maintain hydration, improve nutrition, and oral hygiene

Prevention

- Nonpharmacological
  - Head end elevation
  - Frequent small meals
  - Oral hygiene
  - Restrict tube feeding and improve oral feeding
- Pharmacological
  - Prokinetic agents
  - Angiotensin-converting enzyme inhibitors
  - Treat xerostomia, drooling, and oral candidiasis

complications is 7 days. Empyema and lung abscess need longer duration of antibiotics. If three of the following are met then antibiotics can be stopped: absence of fever, normalization of leukocyte count, decrease in CRP by two-thirds of its peak level, obvious radiological improvement in chest X-ray.[41] Rapid clinicoradiological improvement after an event of aspiration suggests aspiration pneumonitis and mandates discontinuation of antibiotics.

Supportive and Preventive Nonpharmacological Measures

Antibiotic treatment is only a part of the management of AP. Management of nutrition, hydration, oropharyngeal dysphagia and betterment of oral hygiene are essential for recovery of the patient.[39] These measures are also essential in preventing further episodes of AP. "The guiding philosophy with all preventive measures is to enable safe oral feeding while reducing oropharyngeal colonization."

- Head end elevation, tucked in chin posture, frequent small meals, slow and careful swallowing, and dietary modification according to the swallowing disorder should be taught. The speech language pathologist and the dietician are essential members of the rehabilitation team and must be involved early
- Dental evaluation to remove decayed teeth and treatment of periodontal disease should be done. Twice daily oral cleaning improves oral health

- Prolonged tube feeding nasogastric/nasoduodenal or percutaneous entero-gastrostomy tubes promote AP.[39] However, if a swallowing dysfunction is relatively temporary, nasogastric feeding can be done with monitoring of gastric residuals.

Supportive and Preventive Pharmacological Measures

- Prokinetics agents can be reduced gastroesophageal reflux
- Oro-pharyngo-esophageal candidiasis must be sought and treated
- Xerostomia can be treated with artificial saliva, pilocarpine, or xylitol containing products
- Anticholinergic medications reduce saliva production in patients with drooling
- Prophylactic measures for peptic ulcer and venous thrombosis
- Cough promoting measures: Angiotensin-converting enzyme (ACE) inhibitors, particularly the lipophilic ACE inhibitors, lead to accumulation of substance P in the upper airways thereby, increasing the sensitivity of the cough reflex. This has shown to have a preventive effect on AP.[42]

CONCLUSION

Aspiration pneumonia is an infectious consequence of aspiration. Oropharyngeal colonization with pathogenic microbiota and swallowing dysfunction due to depressed sensorium or oropharyngeal dysphagia are the two essential requirements for the development of AP. Advanced age, head and neck cancer, neurological disorders, chronic respiratory disorders, and ventilated patients are important risk groups for AP. Signs and symptoms of respiratory decompensation in a patient at risk of aspiration should alert the physician. Gram-negative organisms such as *H. influenzae, Klebsiella, Enterobacter, E. coli* play a more important role than anaerobic organisms. Nevertheless, anaerobic infections must be suspected when a definite history of aspiration occurs in patients with poor oral hygiene or chronic alcoholism or when necrotizing lung disease develops. Apart from antibiotic measures for improving nutrition, hydration, oral hygiene, and swallowing are important.

ACKNOWLEDGMENTS

We are very grateful to Dr Aparna Irodi, Professor, Department of Radiodiagnosis, CMC Vellore, for providing us with the radiology images for the article.

Editor's Comment

Aspiration pneumonia usually refers to an infection caused by less virulent bacteria, primarily anaerobes, a common constituent of the normal flora, in a host prone to aspiration. Aspiration pneumonia (AP) is the pulmonary consequences resulting from the abnormal entry of fluid, particulate exogenous substances, or endogenous secretions into the lower airways. Advanced age, head and neck cancer, neurological disorders, chronic respiratory disorders and ventilated patients are at risk for AP. Nocturnal aspiration is reported to cause recurrent aspiration pneumonitis in 10% of all untreated patients in the above group. Pulmonary complications due to nocturnal aspirations of esophageal contents in achalasia with radiologic evidence of pulmonary damage are also described. There are usually two requirements to produce AP—oropharyngeal colonization with pathogenic gram-negative, gram-positive, and anaerobic microbiota and swallowing dysfunction due to depressed sensorium or oropharyngeal dysphagia—which are the two essential requirements for the development of AP. Mycobacterium fortuitum resistant to most antibiotics may produce pulmonary infection by growing in a fatty supernatant fluid retained in the esophagus. Pulmonary sequelae depend upon the volume and contents of the inoculum and host defense mechanisms. In this article, authors have exhaustively discussed various causes, clinical features, diagnostic methods, and treatment of AP.

Ravindran Chetambath

REFERENCES

1. Marik PE. Pulmonary aspiration syndromes. *Curr Opin Pulm Med.* 2011;17(3):148-54.
2. Mascitti KB, Manaker S, Rohrbach J, et al. Limitations in using aspiration pneumonia as a quality measure. *Infect Control Hosp Epidemiol.* 2009;30(12):1233-5.
3. Mylotte JM, Goodnough S, Naughton BJ. Pneumonia versus aspiration pneumonitis in nursing home residents: Diagnosis and management. *J Am Geriatr Soc.* 2003;51(1):17-23.
4. Marik PE. Aspiration pneumonitis and aspiration pneumonia. *N Engl J Med.* 2001;344(9):665-71.
5. Luk JK, Chan DK. Preventing aspiration pneumonia in older people: Do we have the "know-how"? Hong Kong Med J Xianggang Yi Xue Za Zhi. 2014;20(5):421-7.
6. Bynum LJ, Pierce AK. Pulmonary aspiration of gastric contents. *Am Rev Respir Dis.* 1976;114(6):1129-36.
7. Joundi RA, Wong BM, Leis JA. Antibiotics "just-in-case" in a patient with aspiration pneumonitis. *JAMA* Intern Med. 2015;175(4):489-90.
8. Sukumaran M, Granada MJ, Berger HW, et al. Evaluation of corticosteroid treatment in aspiration of gastric contents: A controlled clinical trial. *Mt Sinai J Med N Y.* 1980;47(4):335-40.
9. Hu X, Yi ES, Ryu JH. Diffuse aspiration bronchiolitis: Analysis of 20 consecutive patients. *J Bras Pneumol.* 2015;41(2):161-6.
10. Cardasis JJ, MacMahon H, Husain AN. The spectrum of lung disease due to chronic occult aspiration. *Ann Am Thorac Soc.* 2014;11(6):865-73.
11. Prather AD, Smith TR, Poletto DM, et al. Aspiration-related lung diseases. *J Thorac Imaging.* 2014;29(5):304-9.

12. Burkett A, Coffey N, Voduc N. Diffuse pulmonary ossification as a rare cause of interstitial lung disease. *Can Respir J.* 2014;21(1):23-4.
13. Betancourt SL, Martinez-Jimenez S, Rossi SE, et al. Lipoid pneumonia: Spectrum of clinical and radiologic manifestations. *AJR Am J Roentgenol.* 2010;194(1):103-9.
14. Almirall J, Cabré M, Clavé P. Complications of oropharyngeal dysphagia: Aspiration pneumonia. *Nestle Nutr Inst Workshop Ser.* 2012;72:67-76.
15. Ebihara S, Sekiya H, Miyagi M, et al. Dysphagia, dystussia, and aspiration pneumonia in elderly people. *J Thorac Dis.* 2016;8(3):632-9.
16. van der Maarel-Wierink CD, Vanobbergen JNO, Bronkhorst EM, et al. Risk factors for aspiration pneumonia in frail older people: A systematic literature review. *J Am Med Dir Assoc.* 2011;12(5):344-54.
17. van der Maarel-Wierink CD, Vanobbergen JN, Bronkhorst EM, et al. Meta-analysis of dysphagia and aspiration pneumonia in frail elders. *J Dent Res.* 2011;90(12):1398-404.
18. Denaro N, Merlano MC, Russi EG. Dysphagia in head and neck cancer patients: Pretreatment evaluation, predictive factors, and assessment during radio-chemotherapy, recommendations. *Clin Exp Otorhinolaryngol.* 2013;6(3):117-26.
19. Kawai S, Yokota T, Onozawa Y, et al. Risk factors for aspiration pneumonia after definitive chemoradiotherapy or bio-radiotherapy for locally advanced head and neck cancer: a monocentric case control study. *BMC* Cancer. 2017;17(1):59.
20. Chu CN, Muo CH, Chen SW, et al. Incidence of pneumonia and risk factors among patients with head and neck cancer undergoing radiotherapy. *BMC Cancer.* 2013;13:370.
21. Mortensen HR, Jensen K, Grau C. Aspiration pneumonia in patients treated with radiotherapy for head and neck cancer. *Acta Oncol.* 2013;52(2):270-6.
22. Armstrong JR, Mosher BD. Aspiration pneumonia after stroke: Intervention and prevention. *Neurohospitalist.* 2011;1(2):85-93.
23. Hannawi Y, Hannawi B, Rao CPV, et al. Stroke-associated pneumonia: Major advances and obstacles. Cerebrovasc *Dis Basel Switz.* 2013;35(5):430-43.
24. Brogan E, Langdon C, Brookes K, et al. Dysphagia and factors associated with respiratory infections in the first week post stroke. *Neuroepidemiology.* 2014;43(2):140-4.
25. Westendorp WF, Nederkoorn PJ, Vermeij JD, et al. Post-stroke infection: A systematic review and meta-analysis. *BMC Neurol.* 2011;11:110.
26. Mehanna R, Jankovic J. Respiratory problems in neurologic movement disorders. *Parkinsonism Relat Disord.* 2010;16(10):628-38.
27. Erasmus CE, van Hulst K, Rotteveel JJ, et al. Clinical practice: swallowing problems in cerebral palsy. *Eur J Pediatr.* 2012;171(3):409-14.
28. Gerdung CA, Tsang A, Yasseen AS, et al. Association between chronic aspiration and chronic airway infection with pseudomonas aeruginosa and other gram-negative bacteria in children with cerebral palsy. *Lung.* 2016;194(2):307-14.
29. Japanese Respiratory Society. Ventilator-associated pneumonia. *Respirol Carlton Vic.* 2009;14 (Suppl 2): S51-58.
30. El-Solh AA, Pietrantoni C, Bhat A, et al. Microbiology of severe aspiration pneumonia in institutionalized elderly. *Am J Respir Crit Care Med.* 2003;167(12):1650-4.
31. Pace CC, McCullough GH. The association between oral microorgansims and aspiration pneumonia in the institutionalized elderly: Review and recommendations. *Dysphagia.* 2010;25(4):307-22.
32. Hospital-acquired pneumonia in adults: diagnosis, assessment of severity, initial antimicrobial therapy, and preventive strategies. A consensus statement, American Thoracic Society, November 1995. *Am J Respir Crit Care Med.* 1996;153(5):1711-25.
33. Teramoto S, Yoshida K, Hizawa N. Update on the pathogenesis and management of pneumonia in the elderly-roles of aspiration pneumonia. *Respir Investig.* 2015;53(5):178-84.
34. Skull SA, Andrews RM, Byrnes GB, et al. Hospitalized community-acquired pneumonia in the elderly: An Australian case-cohort study. *Epidemiol Infect.* 2009;137(2):194-202.

35. El-Solh AA, Vora H, Knight PR, et al. Diagnostic use of serum procalcitonin levels in pulmonary aspiration syndromes. *Crit Care Med.* 2011;39(6):1251-6.
36. Komiya K, Ishii H, Umeki K, et al. Computed tomography findings of aspiration pneumonia in 53 patients. *Geriatr Gerontol Int.* 2013;13(3):580-5.
37. Brodsky MB, Suiter DM, González-Fernández M, et al. Screening accuracy for aspiration using bedside water swallow tests. *Chest.* 2016;150(1):148-63.
38. Chong MS, Lieu PK, Sitoh YY, et al. Bedside clinical methods useful as screening test for aspiration in elderly patients with recent and previous strokes. *Ann Acad Med Singapore.* 2003;32(6):790-94.
39. Australian and New Zealand Society for Geriatric Medicine. Australian and New Zealand Society for Geriatric Medicine. Position statement - dysphagia and aspiration in older people*. *Australas J Ageing.* 2011;30(2):98-103.
40. Mandell LA, Wunderink RG, Anzueto A, et al. Infectious Diseases Society of America/American Thoracic Society Consensus Guidelines on the Management of Community-Acquired Pneumonia in Adults. *Clin Infect Dis.* 2007;44(Supplement 2):S27-72.
41. Ogasawara T, Umezawa H, Naito Y, et al. Procalcitonin-guided antibiotic therapy in aspiration pneumonia and an assessment of the continuation of oral intake. *Respir Investig.* 2014;52(2):107-13.
42. Shinohara Y, Origasa H. Post-stroke pneumonia prevention by angiotensin-converting enzyme inhibitors: Results of a meta-analysis of five studies in Asians. *Adv Ther.* 2012;29(10):900-12.

World Clin Pulm Crit Care Med. 2019;6(1):198-214.

Pneumonia in Children

[1,*]Sunny A Thomas MD FAAP, [2]Ravindran Chetambath MD DTCD FRCP MBA

[1]Department of Family and Community Medicine, Penn State College of Medicine
Hershey, Pennsylvania, USA
[2]Department of Pulmonary Medicine, DM Wayanad Institute of Medical Sciences
Wayanad, Kerala, India

ABSTRACT

Pneumonia causes substantial morbidity in children worldwide. The incidence of pneumonia is the highest in children under 5 years of age and the number of complicated and severe pneumonia seems to be increasing. If deaths from prematurity and its complications are excluded, the single leading cause of mortality in children under 5 years of age is pneumonia. Burden of pneumonia can be diminished using preventive measures ranging from the simplest infection control methods like hand washing, vaccinations against infections, limiting exposure to infectious cases, and preventing exposure to tobacco smoke.

INTRODUCTION

Pneumonia is one of the leading causes of mortality in children below 5 years of age. In 2015, one out of every six childhood deaths (920,000 deaths per year) were due to pneumonia. There are more than 150 million new episodes of pneumonia each year worldwide and the majority of these are in developing countries especially in the Sub-Saharan Africa and South Asia. World Health Organization (WHO) estimates that pneumonia is responsible for 15% of all deaths in children under 5 years of age which is a decrease from the prior estimates of 19% (Figure 1). Most common pathogens associated with childhood pneumonia are *Streptococcus pneumoniae*, *Haemophilus influenzae*, and many viruses. Major risk factors contributing to the incidence are lack of exclusive breastfeeding, undernutrition, indoor pollution, parental smoking, overcrowded living conditions, and inadequate immunizations. Wide use of vaccines for *Haemophilus influenzae*

*Corresponding author
Email: sathomas60@gmail.com

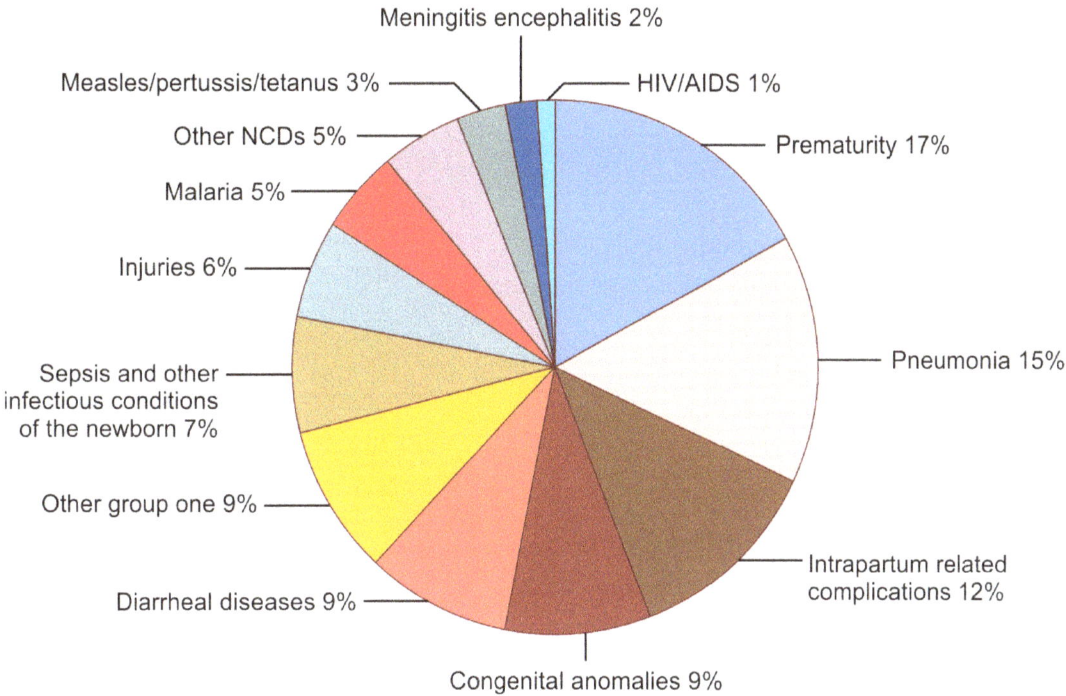

NCDs, non-communicable diseases; HIV, human immunodeficiency virus; AIDS, acquired immune deficiency syndrome.

Figure 1: Cause of death among children less than 5 years of age.

Source: WHO and Maternal and Child Epidemiology Estimation Group (MCEE) estimates 2015 (Reproduced with permission)

type B (HIB), pneumococcus and influenza virus (HIB, PCV 7 and 13, influenza), better diagnostic methods, and availability of better treatments have reduced mortality in developed countries. In spite of documented decrease in number of deaths, burden of the disease remains, as the rest of the world struggles to reduce mortality in children from many infectious diseases including pneumonia.[1-3] This article reviews the etiology, pathophysiology, clinical features, diagnosis, and practical approach to treatment of pneumonia in children.

DEFINITION AND CLASSIFICATION

There is no single definition for pneumonia, that is specific and universally accepted. In many childhood respiratory illnesses, clinical symptoms and signs can overlap. The WHO uses respiratory rate (RR) as an important criteria when defining pneumonia in children. Pneumonia is an infection of the lower respiratory tract usually presenting with fever, cough, tachypnea, evidence of parenchymal involvement on physical examination, and confirmed by radiological findings. The presentation and clinical features can differ in children of each age group. Classification of pneumonia which can help to design appropriate management and selection of treatment can be done in different ways. Based on the anatomical distribution, pneumonia can be lobar, interstitial, or bronchopneumonia. Defined by the origin of infection, pneumonia can be:

- Community-acquired pneumonia (CAP), which refers to an infection acquired outside of a hospital in previously healthy individual
- Hospital-acquired pneumonia (HAP), also called nosocomial infection, occurs when a patient acquires an infection after being in the hospital for two or more days
- Ventilator-associated pneumonia (VAP), which results when a patient on a ventilator develops an infection, often with more resistant and unusual pathogens
- Health care associated pneumonia (HCAP) is another entity when infection is acquired from a long term healthcare facility or a dialysis treatment center.

The pathogens involved in these situations are typically multidrug resistant gram-negative organisms like *Pseudomonas, Enterobacter, Serratia*, and gram-positive cocci such as methicillin-resistant *Staphylococcus aureus*.[4-6]

Aspiration pneumonia is due to aspiration of gastric contents in to the lungs and is seen in children who have compromised gag reflex and those who are semiconscious, comatose, or after anesthesia. Most pathogens involved are anaerobes like gram-positive cocci, *Bacteroides, Fusobacteria*, and aerobic organisms like *Klebsiella, Escherichia coli*, and *Staphylococcus aureus*.

A wide variety of viral and bacterial agents are responsible for pneumonia in children (Table 1). Besides these organisms, there are some fungi and other opportunistic pathogens that can cause pneumonia in children whose immune status is compromised.

RISK FACTORS

Several risk factors have been identified and associated with increased incidence for pneumonia and its severity. The environmental risk factors include overcrowding, indoor pollutants from use of biomass fuels, environmental tobacco smoke, and day care attendance. Other factors are malnutrition, lower socioeconomic status, lack of exclusive breastfeeding, child with compromised immune system or underlying lung disease, inadequate accessibility to health care, and lack of immunizations.[7,8]

PATHOPHYSIOLOGY

Normally, physiological defense mechanisms of the respiratory tract prevent organisms from reaching the lungs and cause inflammation. These are the normal

Table 1: Pathogens Causing Pneumonia in Different Age Groups

Etiology of pneumonia based on age

Age group	Bacterial pathogens	Viral pathogens
Neonates	• Group B *Streptococcus* • Gram-negative bacilli • *Listeria monocytogenes* • *Streptococcus pneumoniae* • *Bordetella pertussis* • *Chlamydia trachomatis* • *Ureaplasma urealyticum* • Anaerobes • Other agents: Toxoplasma	• Respiratory syncytial virus • Influenza • Parainfluenza • Human metapneumovirus • Herpes simplex • Cytomegalovirus • Mumps • Congenital rubella
Infants and young children	• *Streptococcus pneumoniae* • *Mycoplasma pneumoniae* • *Staphylococcus aureus* • Group A *Streptococcus* • *Haemophilus influenzae* type B • *Chlamydia trachomatis* • *Mycobacterium tuberculosis* • *Bordetella pertussis* • *Ureaplasma urealyticum*	• Respiratory syncytial virus • Influenza • Parainfluenza • Human metapneumovirus
Children and adolescents	• *Streptococcus pneumoniae* • *Staphylococcus aureus* • Group A *Streptococcus* • *Haemophilus influenzae* type B • *Moraxella catarrhalis* • *Mycobacterium tuberculosis* • *Legionella*	• Influenza • Parainfluenza • Adenovirus • Epstein–Barr virus • Human metapneumovirus • Human bocavirus

cough reflex, mucociliary action of the lining cells of the respiratory tract, and immunologic agents like secretory immunoglobulin A (IgA), macrophages in the bronchioles, and alveoli. Viral pneumonia usually begins with the onset of an upper respiratory tract infection resulting from exposure to an infected individual through cough, sneezing, or fomites. Once the organism reaches the lower respiratory tract, infected epithelium loses ciliary function, loses shape and begins to slough off into the smaller airways. As a result of this inflammatory edema, airway obstruction occur leading to ventilation-perfusion mismatch and hypoxemia. Complete obstruction of the airways cause distal atelectasis.

Bacterial pathogens that cause pneumonia are usually colonized in the nasopharynx, and then gain access to the lungs by aspiration or hematological spread. Virulence of the organism, absence of specific immunity, and a preceding viral infection of the respiratory tract will result in infection. Inflammatory response by the bacterial pathogens with sloughing of cells and excessive mucus will cause airway obstruction.

Streptococcus pneumoniae produces local edema and proliferation of the organism that spreads to adjacent portion of the lung. This results in the characteristic lobar pneumonia described in four stages.

1. Congestion: The first stage (days 1–2) starts with vascular engorgement and partial obstruction of lung parenchyma with serous exudate, bacteria and neutrophils in the alveoli
2. Red hepatization: In the second stage (days 3–4), the affected lung appears to be reddish, similar to the consistency of liver, showing hyperemia and mucosal edema, deposition of fibrin, and infiltration of the alveoli by polymorphonuclear leukocytes
3. Gray hepatization: In the third stage (days 5–7) lung becomes gray brown because of fibrinopurulent exudate, red cell disintegration, and hemosiderin macrophage activity
4. Resolution: The final stage (days 8–21) occurs with phagocytosis of the fibrinous material by the macrophages and clearing with restoration of the normal pulmonary architecture.

Streptococcus pneumoniae may cause bronchopneumonia with extensive areas of hemorrhagic necrosis, irregular areas of cavitation of the lung parenchyma and may develop into pneumatoceles and empyema.

Group A *Streptococcus* causes diffuse infection with interstitial pneumonia, with extension into interalveolar septa and pleural involvement.

Mycoplasma pneumoniae after attaching to the respiratory epithelium inhibits mucociliary action leading to cellular destruction and inflammatory response leading to edema and airway obstruction.[9-12]

CLINICAL FEATURES

Clinical symptoms can vary in each age group with regard to their presentation. It is difficult to clinically distinguish between bacterial and viral pneumonia. A preceding upper respiratory infection, followed by high fever and cough may be seen with bacterial pneumonia. In all age groups the most common presenting symptoms are fever, cough, and tachypnea. In neonates, fever may not always be a reliable sign but they can present with irritability, poor feeding, and breathing difficulties. Older children may present with the classical symptoms. Grunting, nasal flaring, and retractions are often seen in severe cases of pneumonia. In the early stages, only intercostal retractions are seen, but as disease progresses, supraclavicular retractions and "head bobbing" can be noticed.[13]

Table 2: Respiratory Rate as a Marker of Severity of Pneumonia	
Age in months	**Respiratory rate**
Less than 2 months	>60 breaths/min
2–12 months	>50 breaths/min
1–5 years	>40 breaths/min
>5 years	>30 breaths/min

Tachypnea

It is considered as a consistent feature of pneumonia. The WHO uses the RR to identify children with pneumonia as radiological services are not readily available in many areas (Table 2). The following are upper limits considered for tachypnea in children with pneumonia. Absence of tachypnea can be used as a negative sign to rule out significant lower respiratory tract illness.[14]

Grunting

Infants with lower respiratory tract disease will show grunting in an attempt to keep the smaller airways open by increasing the positive end expiratory pressure.

Cyanosis

Even though not a sensitive indicator in very young infants, children can develop cyanosis in the presence of pneumonia. Pulse oximetry is used to measure the oxygenation status.

Auscultation Findings

In early stages of pneumonia, auscultation shows decreased breath sounds on affected side. In the later stages, crackles and rhonchi can become evident. With onset of consolidation, dullness is noted on percussion.

DIAGNOSIS

The diagnosis of pneumonia is based on history, physical examination, and radiological confirmation. Children who have mild symptoms are not candidates for hospitalization and do not require a chest X-ray to initiate treatment. Pneumonia is usually diagnosed if there is X-ray opacification on the background of suggestive symptoms (Figure 2). X-ray chest often shows opacification with air

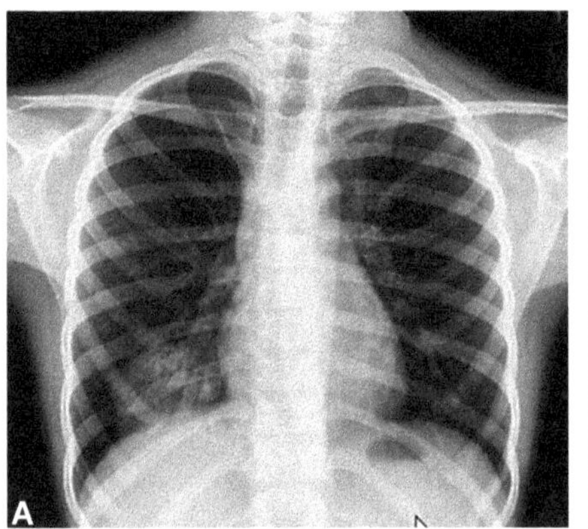
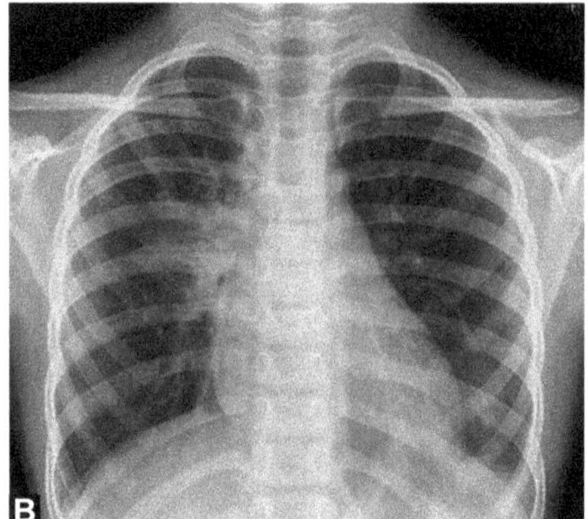

Figure 2: A, X-ray of an 8-year-old girl with segmental pneumonia right lower lobe; **B,** X-ray of a 6-year-old girl with bronchiectasis showing the right upper lobe consolidation.

bronchogram, patchy infiltrates, subsegmental atelectasis, or pneumatocele. In a study published in 2006, most children diagnosed with nonsevere pneumonia on the basis of WHO definition had normal chest radiographs.[15]

Lung ultrasound is being used as another noninvasive method for diagnosing pneumonia. There is high accuracy in the interpretation and can be substituted for chest X-rays especially in countries where radiological services are limited.[16]

Pulse oximetry is useful to assess degree of hypoxemia which, when present increases risk of death caused by pneumonia.

Blood tests are not routinely needed for outpatient management of pneumonia and they often do not help to differentiate bacterial from viral pneumonia. Complete blood count, erythrocyte sedimentation rate, and C-reactive protein may be useful in hospitalized children to monitor response to treatment.

Microbiological tests can help to determine the causative agent, but are not always practical. Less invasive methods like sputum Gram stain and acid-fast bacilli smear can be useful in identifying some of the causative organisms. Culture of sputum and blood has limited values in the early outpatient management.

Invasive studies such as nasopharyngeal swabs, tracheal aspirate, and bronchial washings for viral detection by polymerase chain reaction (PCR) or immunofluorescence are used when severity of the disease warrants identification of the specific agents involved. Pleural fluid culture will have poor yield as most children would have received antibiotics before any aspiration is done.

Nasopharyngeal samples offer rapid identification with polymerase chain reaction techniques to detect several pathogens like respiratory syncytial virus, influenza, *Bordetella pertussis*, and *Mycoplasma*.

Blood culture is not routinely done as the yield is low in nontoxic and immunized children, but useful in hospitalized patients.

Serological tests for detecting pneumococcal antibody are complex and not recommended for routine use. However, urinary antigen detection for *S. pneumoniae* and *Legionella* has some clinical use as negative predictors. Polymerase chain reaction can be used to detect atypical pathogens causing pneumonia. Direct fluorescent antibody and complement fixation tests are used for the detection of *Legionella, Chlamydia, Mycoplasma*, and histoplasmosis. Antigen detection in serum can be used for *Cryptococcus*.[16-18]

Tuberculin skin tests (Mantoux) or interferon-gamma release assay (IGRAs QuantiFERON-TB Gold) can be done when exposure is suspected.[19]

MANAGEMENT

Management of pneumonia has to be individualized based on the age of the patient and clinical presentation (Figure 3). Immunization status, past history of repeated infections, and use of antibiotics are to be considered when making treatment decisions. Most children who are immunologically sound presenting

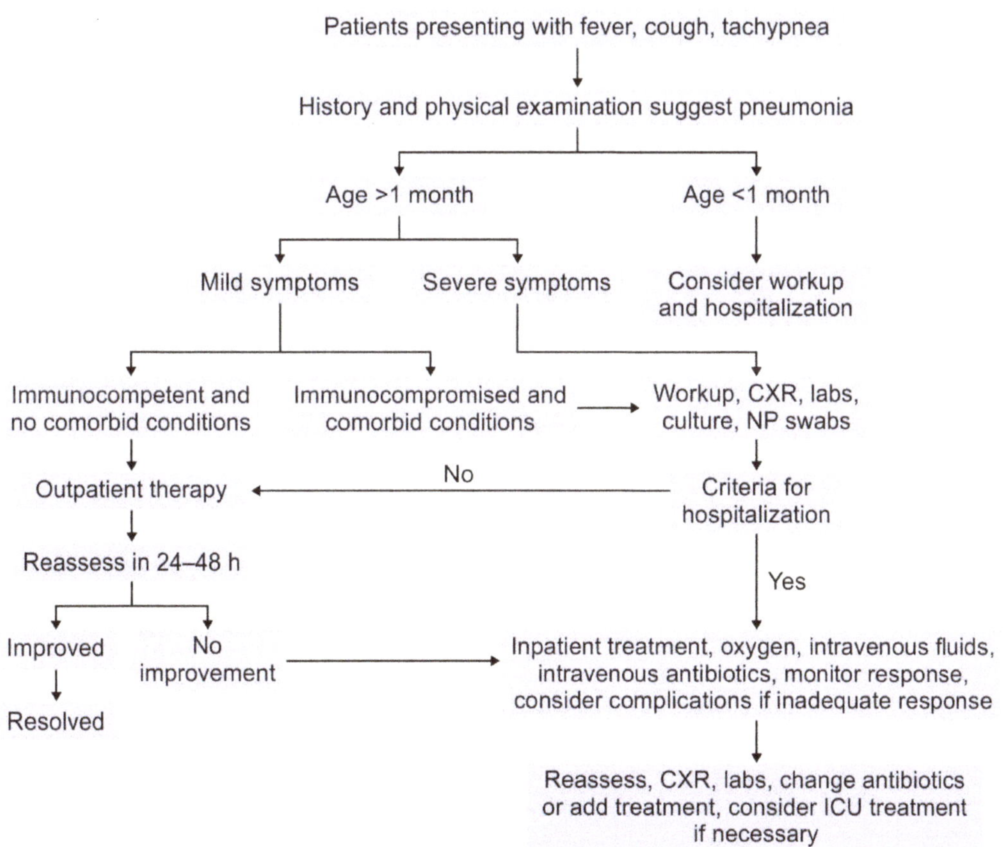

CXR, chest X-ray; NP, nasopharyngeal; IV, intravenous; ICU, intensive care unit.

Figure 3: Algorithm for practical approach to management of pneumonia in children.

with mild to moderate symptoms can be treated as outpatients. Management of dehydration is universally recommended. Even the auscultation and radiological findings can be misleading when there is dehydration. Since the causative organism is not always identified, empirical treatment with antibiotics is the key point in treating bacterial pneumonia (Table 3). Amoxicillin in appropriate dose (90 mg/kg/day) is the first line therapy for most children (Table 4). For those with allergy to amoxicillin, a cephalosporin or macrolide can be chosen. For older children and adolescents, atypical pathogens are likely and treatment with macrolide (azithromycin or clarithromycin) is considered.[20-22]

Indications for Hospitalization

Most cases of pneumonia can be managed in the outpatient setting. Those patients presenting with severe symptoms are evaluated for hospitalization and inpatient management. The following criteria are generally considered for hospitalization:

- Hypoxemia (oxygen saturation <92%)
- Infants younger than 3–6 months
- Signs of respiratory distress: Tachypnea—RR more than 60 breaths/min in infants less than 12 months, RR more than 50 breaths/min in children, grunting, intercostal retractions, difficulty breathing, and apnea at any age
- Signs of dehydration—poor capillary refill
- Vomiting and inability to maintain hydration
- Patients with comorbid conditions (cardiac, genetic, and metabolic conditions)
- Patients with sickle cell and other immunocompromised states
- Failed outpatient therapy or suspected complications
- Inability of primary care takers to successfully manage sick patients
- Intensive care management is needed for patients with severe respiratory distress requiring endotracheal intubation and ventilator support and those with hypotension and altered mental status.[23,24]

Table 3: Common Agents Used for Treating Pneumonia in Children

Age group	First line	Alternate selection	Additional medications	Antiviral medications
Neonates	Ampicillin and gentamicin	Ampicillin Cefotaxime		Acyclovir
Infants and Preschool	Amoxicillin	Amoxicillin/clavulanate Cephalosporins	Azithromycin Clarithromycin	Oseltamivir
School age and above	Amoxicillin	Amoxicillin/clavulanate Cephalosporins Levofloxacin	Azithromycin Clarithromycin	Oseltamivir

Table 4: Antibiotic Dosage and Intervals for Each Age Group

Medication	Age/weight	Dose(mg/kg/day)	Interval hours	Route
Amoxicillin		90	12	PO (high dose)
Amoxicillin/clavulanate		90	12	PO
Ampicillin+Sulbactum	Infants	100–150 (infants) 100–200 (child)	6	IM/IV
Azithromycin		10 mg/kg 5 mg/kg	Day 1 Day 2–5	PO/(IV available)
Cefdinir		14	24	PO
Cefuroxime		30 75–150	12 8	PO IV
Clarithromycin		15	12	PO
Clindamycin		30 25–40	8 12	PO IM/IV
Ceftriaxone		50–100	12	IM/IV
Co-Trimoxazole	Not for <2 months	20	6–8	PO/IV
Doxycycline	<45kg >45 kg	2.2 mg/kg/dose 100 mg/dose	12 12	PO/IV PO/IV
Erythromycin		30–40	6	PO
Linezolid Linezolid	Up to 11 years Over 12 years	10 mg/kg/dose 600 mg/dose	8 12	IV/PO
Levofloxacin		10 mg/kg (up to a maximum of 500 mg/day	24	PO/IV
Penicillin G Aqueous Penicillin A Benzathine		100,000–400,000 U/kg/day 1.2 million U/dose	6 24	IM/IV IM ONLY
Vancomycin		40–60	6	IV

PO, per oral; IV, intravenous; IM, intramuscular.

COMPLICATIONS

With appropriate treatment, symptoms of fever, tachypnea, hypoxemia, and poor appetite begins to improve but resolution of the consolidation is a slower process. Failure to improve after optimal therapy is an indication for further evaluation to exclude complications. The complications are more pronounced in bacterial than viral infections.[25,26]

Possible Complications

- Pleural effusion
- Empyema
- Pneumatocele
- Pneumothorax
- Pneumomediastinum
- Necrotizing pneumonia
- Lung abscess
- Sepsis.

Pleural Effusion and Empyema

Presence of exudative fluid (pleural effusion) and pus (empyema) within the pleural space are frequent complications of pneumonia. Most common agents are *Streptococcus pneumoniae, Streptococcus pyogenes, Staphylococcus aureus*, and *Mycobacterium tuberculosis*. Plain chest X-rays, ultrasound, or chest CT scans are useful in diagnosis. Small pleural effusions do not require any active treatment, but moderate to large effusions and empyema may need aspiration or chest tube drainage. More serious cases may require video assisted thoracoscopic surgery and decortication and use of fibrinolytics.

Necrotizing Pneumonia

It is an uncommon complication of pneumonia in children and is characterized by liquefaction and cavitation of pulmonary tissue. The most frequently associated pathogen is *Streptococcus pneumoniae*, especially serotypes 3 and 14. Other pathogens involved include group A streptococci, *Staphylococcus aureus,* and *Mycoplasma pneumoniae*. Chest CT scans are useful in the diagnosis. Treatment includes prolonged intravenous antibiotics and pleural drainage if complicated with empyema.

Lung Abscess

Primary lung abscesses are caused by aspirations that occur in neurologically intact patient and secondary lung abscesses are seen in neurologically compromised patients and those with any congenital lung anomaly. Pathogens identified in lung abscess are aerobes, anaerobes, and fungi. In many cases, polymicrobial pathogens are present. *Staphylococcus aureus* and *Streptococcus pneumoniae* are the major isolates along with gram-negative bacilli. The common symptoms in children who develop lung abscess are fever, cough, tachypnea, chest pain, sputum production with hemoptysis, and weight loss. Diagnosis is mainly with chest X-rays, but CT scan always is recommended. Treatment involves high dose intravenous antibiotics (penicillin, ampicillin plus sulbactam, or amoxicillin plus clavulanic acid), third generation cephalosporins, aminoglycosides, and clindamycin. Immunocompromised patients may need consideration for antifungal agents. Failure to improve persistent fevers after antibiotics for over 7 days are indications for drainage procedures.[27,28]

Fungal Pneumonia in Children

Due to the widespread use of broad spectrum antibiotics, cytotoxic drugs, and systemic corticosteroids, incidence and clinical significance of fungal infection in children are increasing. Fungi that cause pneumonia in children can be opportunistic and endemic pathogens. Main organisms causing fungal pneumonia are *Aspergillus* species, *Candida* species, *Histoplasma capsulatum, Coccidioides* species, *Blastomyces dermatitidis*, and *Cryptococcus neoformans.*

Risk factors for development of fungal pneumonia are prematurity, malnutrition, diseases that affect immune function such as leukemia, agranulocytosis and aplastic anemia, metabolic disorders such as diabetes and renal failure, use of corticosteroids and other immunosuppressive drugs, congenital immune deficiency, and acquired immune deficiency syndrome.

Diagnosis is by microscopic identification and isolation of the fungi from bronchoalveolar lavage (BAL). An enzyme linked immunosorbent assay test from serum or BAL fluid is also found to be useful in children. In difficult cases, percutaneous or open lung biopsy specimen is obtained for culture and histopathological examination.

Antifungal agents used in children are itraconazole, fluconazole, voriconazole, and liposomal amphotericin B.[29-31]

Pneumonia in Immunocompromised Children

Immunocompromised patients present great challenge with regard to diagnosis and management. Even common pathogens can present with severe symptoms and show inadequate response to treatment. Secondary immune deficiencies are caused by immunosuppressive drugs, infections (human immunodeficiency virus), and malnutrition. Cellular immunodeficiency makes the patient susceptible to pathogens like *Mycobacterium tuberculosis*, and opportunistic pathogens like *Pneumocystis jirovecii*, *Cytomegalovirus*, and *Candida* species. Humoral immunodeficiency can result in recurrent infections with encapsulated bacteria including *Streptococcus pneumoniae* and *Haemophilus influenzae.* Immune deficiency from phagocytic cell dysfunction can cause recurrent infections with *Staphylococcus aureus, Serratia, Aspergillus* and *Candida* species.

Neonatal Pneumonia

Pneumonia in neonates often presents with irritability, poor feeding, respiratory distress, retractions, and apnea. Fever when present can be helpful in the diagnosis, but may not be always present. In premature babies with underlying hyaline membrane disease, pneumonia can cause high mortality. Most common pathogens in the newborn are group B *Streptococcus*, *E. coli, S. aureus, Listeria monocytogenes*, and *C. trachomatis* (Table 5). Newborns that develop transient tachypnea of the new born have features that are indistinguishable from those with meconium aspiration syndrome or a group B streptococcal pneumonia. Pathogens causing pneumonia can be acquired during antenatal, perinatal, or postnatal periods.[32-34]

When pneumonia is suspected, initial screening tests includes complete blood count, blood cultures, and radiological examination (Figure 4). Since the symptoms are atypical, CT thorax may be needed to make a confidential diagnosis and to rule out other underlying abnormalities in the respiratory system (Figure 5).

Supportive treatment with oxygen and fluid management are to be initiated in the hospital. Ampicillin and gentamicin are the initial choice for empirical treatment. Once etiology is established definitive treatment should be started. Common agents used to treat neonatal pneumonia are given in table 6.

Table 5: Pathogens Causing Pneumonia in Neonates

When acquired	Bacteria	Virus
Prenatal	• *Listeria monocytogenes* • *Mycobacterium tuberculosis* • *Treponema pallidum*	• Rubella • Varicella zoster • *Cytomegalovirus* • Human immunodeficiency virus • Herpes simplex
Perinatal	• Group B streptococci • Gram-negative (*E. coli, Klebsiella*)	• *Cytomegalovirus* • Herpes simplex
Postnatal	• *Staphylococcus aureus* • *Pseudomonas aeruginosa*	• *Cytomegalovirus* • Herpes simplex • Influenza • Parainfluenza • Respiratory syncytial virus

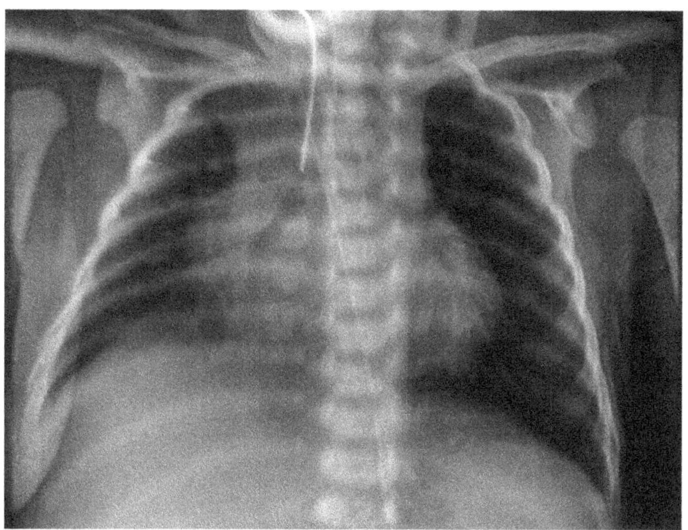

Figure 4: X-ray of 30-day-old baby with laryngomalacia.

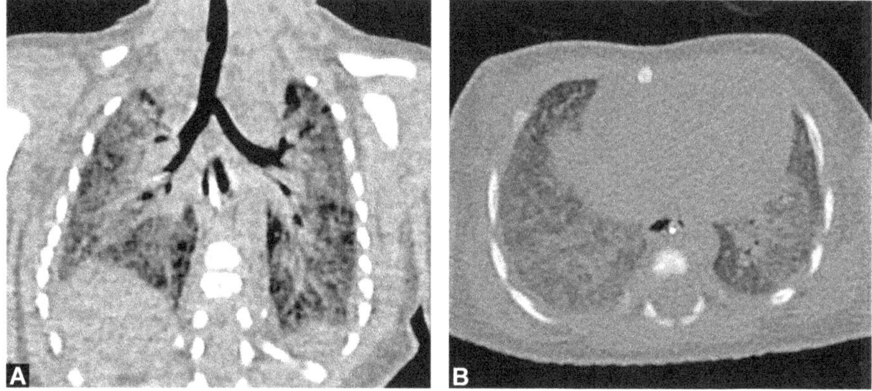

Figure 5: Computed tomography of thorax showing severe pneumonia in a 30-day-old baby with laryngomalacia.

PREVENTION

Immunization against many pathogens like *H. influenzae* type B, *S. pneumoniae*, pertussis, measles, and influenza virus has reduced incidence of pneumonia and hospital admissions in countries where these are implemented. In spite of the proven benefits, there are refusal and opposition to the use of vaccines. Not only is more education needed to dispel myths and eliminate fears about immunizations, but ensuring availability of vaccines and health care support is also needed. The Patient Centered Medical Home is a model that provides consistent medical care to the patients in the area where it is implemented. Establishing a "medical home" for the children will ensure continuity of care that will impact

Table 6: Recommended Medication Dosages for Treatment of Pneumonia in Neonates

Medication	Age/weight range	Dose (mg/kg/day)	Interval hours	Route
Ampicillin		100	12	IM/IV
Cefotaxime	<7 days, <2,000 g	100	12	IM/IV
	>2,000 g	150	8	IV
	>7 days	150	8	
Erythromycin		50	6	PO/(IV available)
Gentamicin	<7 days	5	48	IM/IV
	8–28 days	4	36	
	>29 days	4	24	
Vancomycin	<7 days <1.2 kg	15	24	IV
	1.2-2 kg	10–15	12–18	IV
	>2 kg	10–15	8–12	IV
Acyclovir		30	8	IV

PO, per oral; IV, intravenous; IM, intramuscular.

in reducing mortality rates. Since HIB conjugate vaccines became available in 1990, *Haemophilus* is not a major bacterial pathogen causing pneumonia. With availability of 7 valent pneumococcal conjugate vaccine (PCV7) in 2000 and PCV13 in 2010, the incidence of pneumonia caused by these pathogens have decreased significantly. Influenza vaccine for children older than 6 months has reduced hospitalization rates and is an important preventive strategy. It is also recommended that parents and family members of infants more than 6 months of age should be immunized with influenza and pertussis vaccine to protect the infants from exposure. Reducing smoking and indoor pollution, addressing overcrowding, and promoting exclusive breastfeeding are other factors to prevent pneumonia. Overtreatment with antimicrobials and development of resistance has been a concern in many parts of the world. At the same time, inadequate treatment and delay in seeking medical care has negative impact resulting in higher mortality. Developing better evaluation criteria, judicious use of antimicrobials, encouraging immunizations, reducing indoor pollution, and managing malnutrition will all lead to better outcome and decrease mortality in children.

CONCLUSION

Pneumonia continues to be a leading cause of mortality in children. There are many challenges that need to be addressed to reduce the impact of the disease.

Malnutrition and inadequate access to health care and lack of immunizations are significant factors. Measures to decrease and eliminate child deaths should focus on controlling and managing infectious causes. Developing universally applicable criteria about definition, diagnosis, and management of pneumonia in children can be helpful in standardizing the approach to this problem.

Editor's Comment

Pneumonia in children is often a serious illness and a leading causes of mortality in children less than 5 years of age. In the absence of recognizable signs, fever, cough, and increased respiratory rate are considered important criteria for diagnosis. Etiologically, pneumonias in children are commonly of viral or bacterial origin but may not be clinically distinguishable. It is important to start early treatment for prevention of serious complications and mortality from the illness. Most cases can be managed in the outpatient setting. Hospitalization may be required for those patients presenting with severe symptoms.

Malnutrition, inadequate access to healthcare, and lack of immunizations are important factors of poor prognosis.

Surinder K Jindal

REFERENCES

1. Rudan I, Boschi-Pinto C, Biloglav Z, et al. Epidemiology and etiology of childhood pneumonia. *Bull World Health Organ.* 2008;86(5):408-16.
2. World Health Organization. Pneumonia: Fact Sheet 2016. Available from: http://www.who.int/mediacentre/factsheets/fs331/en/. [Accessed May 04, 2017].
3. Ending Preventable Child Deaths from Pneumonia and Diarrhoea by 2025. 2013. Available from: https://data.unicef.org/wp-content/uploads/2016/11/Ending-Preventable-Child-Deaths-from-Pneumonia-and Diarrhoea-by-2025.pdf. [Accessed May 07, 2017].
4. Scott JA, Wonodi CB, Moisi JC, et al. The definition of pneumonia, the assessment of severity, and clinical standardization in the Pneumonia Etiology Research for Child Health Study. *Clin Infect Dis.* 2012;54(Suppl 2):109-16.
5. Sandora TJ. Hospital epidemiology and infection control for children: Report from the Society for Healthcare Epidemiology of America Pediatric Leadership Council. *J Pediatric Infect Dis Soc.* 2014;3(1):4-6.
6. Chetambath R. Pneumonia. In: Pediatric respiratory illnesses. 2nd ed. New Delhi: Macmillan Medical Communications; 2011. pp. 105-13.
7. Wonodi CB, Deloria-Knoll M, Feikin DR, et al. Evaluation of risk factors for severe pneumonia in children: The Pneumonia Etiology Research for Child Health Study. *Clin Infect Dis.* 2012;54(S2):124-31.
8. Grant CC, Emery D, Milne T, et al. Risk factors for community-acquired pneumonia in pre-school-aged children. *J Paediatr Child Health.* 2011;48(5):402-12.
9. Byington CL, Bradley JS. Pediatric community-acquired pneumonia. In: Cherry JD, Harrison GJ, Kaplan SL, et al., editors. Feigin and Cherry's textbook of pediatric infectious diseases. 7th ed. Philadelphia, PA: Elsevier/Saunders; 2014. pp. 283-92.

10. Johnson JE, Gonzales RA, Olson SJ, et al. The histopathology of fatal untreated human respiratory syncytial virus infection. *Mod Pathol.* 2007;20(1):108-19.
11. Domachowske JB, Rosenberg HF. Respiratory syncytial virus infection: Immune response, immunopathogenesis, and treatment. *Clin Microbiol Rev.* 1999;12(2):298-309.
12. Kelly MS, Sandora TJ. Community-acquired pneumonia. In: Kliegman RM, Nelson WE, Stanton BF, et al., editors. Nelson textbook of pediatrics. Philadelphia, PA: Elsevier; 2016. pp. 2088-94.
13. Gereige RS, Laufer PM. Pneumonia. *Pediatr Rev.* 2013;34(10):438-56.
14. Rucsoni F, Castegneto M, Gagliardi L. Reference values for respiratory rates in the first 3 years of life. *Pediatrics.* 1994;94:350-55.
15. Hazir TY, Nisar SA, Qazi SF, et al. Chest radiography in children aged 2-59 months diagnosed with non-severe pneumonia as defined by World Health Organization: Descriptive multicenter study in Pakistan. *BMJ.* 2006;333(7569):629-34.
16. Pereda MA, Chavez MA, Hooper-Miele CC, et al. Lung ultrasound for the diagnosis of pneumonia in children: A meta-analysis. *Pediatrics.* 2015;135(4):714-72.
17. Nuutila J, Essa-Matti L. Distinction between bacterial and viral infections. *Curr Opin Infect Dis.* 2007;20(3): 304-10.
18. Rajalakshmi B, Kanungo R, Srinivasan S, et al. Pneumolysin in urine: A rapid antigen detection method to diagnose pneumococcal pneumonia in children. *Indian J Med Microbiol.* 2002;20(4):183-6.
19. Roya-Pabon CL, Perez-Velez CM. Tuberculosis exposure, infection and disease in children: A systematic diagnostic approach. *Pneumonia.* 2016;8:23-41.
20. Harris M, Clark J, Coote N, et al. British Thoracic Society guidelines for the management of community acquired pneumonia in children: Update 2011. *Thorax.* 2011;66(S2):1-23.
21. Saux NL, Robinson JL. Canadian Paediatric Society, Infectious Diseases and Immunization Committee. Uncomplicated pneumonia in healthy Canadian children and youth: Practice points for management. *Pediatr* Child Health. 2015;20(8):441-5.
22. Williams DJ, Shah SS. Community-acquired pneumonia in the conjugate vaccine era. *J Pediatric Infect Dis Soc.* 2012;1(4):314-28.
23. Thomas M, Spencer D. Management and complications of pneumonia. *Pediatr Child Health.* 2011;21(5):207-12.
24. Tam PI. Approach to common bacterial infections. *Pediatr Clin North Am.* 2013;60(2):437-53.
25. Puligandla PS, Laberge JM. Respiratory infections: Pneumonia, lung abscess, and empyema. *Semin Pediatr Surg.* 2008;17(1):42-52.
26. Bazrafshan A, Heydarian F, Hashemzadeh A, et al. Surgical causes in lower respiratory tract infection in children. *Patient Saf Qual Improv.* 2015;3(1):196-7.
27. Spencer DA, Thomas MF. Necrotizing pneumonia in children. *Paediatr Respir Rev.* 2014;15(3):240-5.
28. Yen CC, Tang RB, Chen SJ, et al. Pediatric lung abscess: A retrospective review of 23 cases. *J Microbiol Immunol Infect.* 2004;37(1):45-9.
29. Hirschtick RE, Glassroth J, Jordan MC, et al. Bacterial pneumonia in persons infected with the human immunodeficiency virus. Pulmonary Complications of HIV Infection Study Group. *N Engl J Med.* 1995; 333:845-52.
30. American Academy of Pediatrics. In: Kimberlin DW, Brady MT, Jackson MA, editors. Red Book 2015 Report of the Committee on Infectious Diseases. 30th ed. Elk Grove Village, IL: American Academy of Pediatrics 2015; 240(52):828-35.
31. Montenegro BL, Arnold JC. North American dimorphic fungal infections in children. *Pediatr Rev.* 2010;31(6): 40-8.
32. Kimberlin DW, Acosta EP, Prichard MN, et al. Oseltamivir pharmacokinetics, dosing, and resistance among children aged. *J Infect Dis.* 2013;207:709-20.
33. Reid RJ, Fishman PA, Yu O, et al. Patient-centered medical home demonstration: A prospective, quasi-experimental, before and after evaluation. *Am J Manag Care.* 2009;15(9):e71-87.
34. Nissen M D. Congenital and neonatal pneumonia. *Pediatr Respir Rev.* 2007;8(3):195-203.

WORLD CLINICS
Statement of Purpose

The streams of medicine and surgery are evolving constantly at a rapid pace, creating a need for the healthcare professionals to continuously update their knowledge base and skills. This is necessary to offer their patients the best 'real world' treatment options based on current concepts, status, and trends, reflecting the achievements of evidence-based medicine. This pace of advances in medicine is a compelling reason for the physicians and surgeons to seek information through multiple resources, such as journals, workshops and conferences.

WORLD CLINICS are periodicals of evidence-based reviews proposed as a source of comprehensive, state-of-the art reviews written by experts representing the global academia under the mentorship of an Editor-in-Chief. The comments by the 'Guest Editor' (or Editor-in-Chief) given at the end of each article/chapter would be representative of their clinical experience. Each issue of "WORLD CLINICS Pulmonary and Critical Care Medicine" would focus on a single theme covering topics that are relevant to clinical understanding and decision-making. Each topic would be developed to reflect the current evidence, research, existing guidelines and recommendations as well the clinical experience of experts.

Objectives

- Provide up-to-date reviews on disease management, technique, procedure, or technology.
- Help enhance knowledge and skill for application in clinical practice.
- To aid use of evidence in decision-making for improved patient care.
- To help select best treatment options and overcome treatment challenges.

Target Readers

WORLD CLINICS are meant for practicing physicians, fellows, and postgraduate students, who plan to keep abreast with the current best-evidence clinical practices that are recommended and followed by experts globally.

Periodicity

WORLD CLINICS Pulmonary and Critical Care Medicine will be released with a frequency of two issues in a year.

Themes

Each subject area of WORLD CLINICS will cover themes on any of the following:

1. A disease or a disorder (e.g., Pneumonia) OR
2. An organ or an anatomical region (e.g., Wrist, in WORLD CLINICS Orthopedics) OR
3. A technique or a treatment approach (e.g., Various methods for the treatment of CTEV, in WORLD CLINICS Orthopedics) OR
4. A special population group (e.g., Management of HIV infected children patients in WORLD CLINICS Pediatrics) OR
5. A technology (e.g., 3D Ultrasound in diagnosis of gynecological abnormalities in WORLD CLINICS Obstetrics and Gynecology)

WORLD CLINICS
Manuscript Guidelines for Authors

General Guidelines

- Manuscripts must be typed in double-space including all text, references, tables, and figure legends, and should be sent in a single word file.
- For any copyright work, the necessary permissions must be obtained by the author and sent along with the manuscript. These permissions apply to any borrowed, modified, or adapted text, tables, or figures.
- For any production-quality artwork (images, illustrations, etc.) please see the guidelines under images.
- Acknowledgments or disclosures, if required, should be cited before the references.

Author Credits

- Should be in the first page.
- Each author's name, degree, academic or professional affiliation, city, and state (or country).
- E-mail address, mailing address, and telephone number of each co-author.
- If more than one author, mention the corresponding author.
- Please supply 4–6 keywords which will be used to optimize search results.

Subheads

The format for article's headings and subheadings is as follows:
'A' head: All caps, bold.
'B' head: Title case (upper/lower), bold.
'C' head: Title case (upper/lower), bold, italics.
'D' head: Title case (upper lower), normal, Roman.
'E' head: Sentence case (initial letter capital), italics, run in.

References

- References must be cited sequentially only at the end of the manuscript in the order as they appear in the text.
- Follow the Vancouver style for the references, using the Index Medicus abbreviations for journals that are indexed; if a journal is not indexed, use full name.
- If there are more than six authors, cite first six and add "et al.," e.g., Lacasse Y, Selman M, Costabel U, Dalphin JC, Ando M, Morell F, et al. Clinical diagnosis of hypersensitivity pneumonitis. *Am J Respir Crit Care Med.* 2003;168:952-8.

Images

- There is generally no restriction on number of boxes, tables, or images, but keep them to a minimum necessary.
- A maximum of two hand-drawn illustrations and maximum of two algorithms are allowed.
- Medium for delivery of photographs: Individual TIFF or JPEG files each at a resolution no lower than 300 dpi (118 pixels/cm) when viewed at 100 mm width.
- The images and illustrations can also be in full color.

www.ingramcontent.com/pod-product-compliance
Lightning Source LLC
Chambersburg PA
CBHW040140200326
41458CB00025B/6330

* 9 7 8 9 3 5 2 7 0 4 6 6 8 *